Soul to Soul

A Manual for Compassionate Caregiving

Dr. Carol Kasser
and
Joan Phillips, A.D.C.

Dedication

This book is dedicated to the residents and staffs of the nursing homes and assisted living facilities where we have worked. We have learned much from all of you.

It was written to honor our parents: for Marilyn Kasser, and in loving memory of Arthur Kasser, Midge Murray, Fred and Freda Phillips.

Note: We have used **she** throughout Part I because a disproportionate number of nursing home residents are female.

To order additional copies of this book, contact:
Xlibris Corporation
1-888-795-4274
www.Xlibris.com
Orders@Xlibris.com
54353

Contents

INTRODUCTION

We Baby Boomers are the new sandwich generation. As we approach retirement, and deal with our own financial and health crises, we find ourselves squeezed between the needs of our children and grandchildren, and the demands of frail aging parents. Joan and Carol know this from firsthand experience. Recently Joan accompanied her mother on the journey from good health and independence, to dialysis and life in a nursing home, to death. And an accident in 2007 changed Carol's mother from an independent, working, driving, octogenarian to a wheelchair bound semi-invalid fighting to gain some semblance of independence with a walker.

But we bring much more than personal experience to this book about dealing compassionately with the issues surrounding the care of aging parents. From 1993 to 2008, Joan was the activities director of Gwynned Square Rehabilitation Center, one of the top-rated nursing homes in Pennsylvania. Under Joan's guidance, Gwynned's extensive activities programming and outstanding activities staff attracted the attention of state and national nursing home leaders. Joan presided over a variety of programs for residents with different levels of abilities, including special Alzheimer's programs. She is a member of PAPA (The Pennsylvania Activity Professionals Association). She has served that organization as a member of the Board of Directors, Editor of the PAPA Newsletter, and co-chair of the annual convention. She also belongs to NCCAP (National Certification Council of Activity Professionals) and PTRS(Pennsylvania Therapeutic Recreation Society). She is also a former member of NAAP (National Association of Activity Professionals).

Carol took a different path to expertise in aging. After earning a B.A. in English at the University of Pennsylvania, an M.A. in English Literature from Western Connecticut State University, and an Ed.D. in English Education from Temple University, Dr. Kasser spent twenty years teaching English and ESL at The Community College of Philadelphia. The desire for a mid-life career change sent Carol to Gratz College to get an M.A. in Jewish Studies. She also attended The Reconstructionist Rabbinical College for three years before becoming a geriatric chaplain in 1989. Carol earned certificates in gerontology and pastoral counseling. She also has CPE (Clinical Pastoral Education) training in both hospital and geriatric settings. Dr. Kasser has been a chaplain for the Board of Rabbis of Philadelphia, the Jewish Chaplaincy and Healing Program, and several independent senior care facilities. Because she sometimes served in interfaith settings, she also received an ordination in Interfaith Ministry. Her chaplaincy work led her to write the books *Cast Me Not off When I Am Old, Manna For the Soul,* and *Reflections: Reading of Spirituality, Gratitude and Love.* In addition, she has given lectures and workshops on spirituality and healing, spirituality and aging, and Jewish spirituality for various colleges and religious groups.

Joan and Carol recognize the need for this book to help families in a rapidly aging world. There are an increasing number of octogenarians, nonagenarians and centenarians. According to U.S. government census predictions, by the year 2010, there will be 34,120,000 people aged 65-84 living in the United States. Of these, 6,123,000 will be over age 85. This aging is a mixed blessing. It allows youth to learn from the experience of their elders. It means more children will get to know their grandparents and great-grandparents. But the aging process is also often accompanied by financial problems, housing difficulties, as well as mental and physical limitations. And with this elderly population comes an army of children, many of them senior citizens themselves, who are the caretakers for their aging parents. **Soul to Soul: a Manual for Compassionate Caregiving** is for all of those loving caregivers.

This book aims at facilitating decisions you may have to make about frail, aging parents. We have compiled this advice and these stories based on years of observation and conversation with residents and family members. We hope this information will help you make the difficult decisions that lie ahead. From this book, you will learn how to have meaningful interaction with frail elders, even those with Alzheimer's. In fact, our aim is to show you how to interact soul to soul with your aging parent.

Philosopher Martin Buber spoke about I-it and I-thou relationships. In I-it relationships one person diminishes the other in some way. I-thou relationships are soul to soul encounters. Too often elders, especially those in nursing homes are treated as It. They are called "Sweetie" or "Honey" by people 1/3 their age. They may be infantilized or ignored. Even well-meaning children talk about role reversal, about becoming the parent to their parent.

But the parent is not a child despite a failing physical and mental condition. Talking to a parent as a child does not permit a soul to soul encounter and disregards the commandment "Honor Your Father and Mother."

Both Carol and Joan have had days when they showed unfailing patience with troublesome residents in the nursing home, but were short-tempered with their mothers or spouses over relatively minor issues when they got home.

They learned that they could avoid that annoyed tone of voice, and strive for a soul to soul interaction, when they suspended the emotional baggage that comes in any parent-child or spousal relationship and treated their family member with the same respect and dignity they afforded strangers in the same situation. It is a practice they both highly recommend to all caregivers.

The first section of the book covers warning signs children should look for to indicate that their parents should no longer live alone. It suggests home adaptations and services that may allow frail elders to stay in their homes longer. Finally it gives a complete introduction to the variety of housing options available for the elderly. It concludes with a list of questions to ask when evaluating a facility.

The second section of the book presents a series of vignettes from nursing homes that help family members understand and interact with the elders they love, including those suffering from Alzheimer's or other forms of dementia. The authors suggest concrete activities and methods of communicating so that visits provide the most benefit to the residents and the least stress to the visitors.

This book borrows from Martin-Buber's theory of I-thou encounters. It is our intent to show how to see and encourage the holy in interacting with our elders.

While there are many books on aging, none of them personalize the nursing home residents as the vignettes in this book do. Every reader will recognize something their loved one has said or done in the personal stories told in this book. And each story comes with a discussion of what the resident is trying to communicate and how the family can best respond when they are inevitably confronted with one of these situations.

PART I

When Home Isn't Safe Anymore

There's no place like home.
—Dorothy in the **Wizard of Oz**

---

* *Falls are the leading cause of injury deaths for older Americans.*
* *Half of all falls occur at home.*
* *One-third of adults over 65 and over one-half of adults over 80 fall at least once each year.*

Chapter 1

Signs of Trouble

How do you know when it is time for a family member to consider alternative housing? The vast majority of seniors will not voluntarily make a move from their own home. Because physical and mental decline usually happens slowly, people rarely recognize the descent themselves. They might say, "I don't see as well as I used to" or "My memory is not like it was," but they rarely recognize when their hearing, memory, vision, or reflexes are so impaired that they are a danger to themselves or others.

These are some of the signs that might indicate danger. When they have trouble writing checks, cooking a favorite dish, operating a commonly-used appliance, pay attention. Sometimes confusion can be a sign of improper nutrition, poor hydration, or misuse of medication. But it can also be a sign of a mini-stroke or the onset of Alzheimer's. In all of these cases, timely medical intervention is crucial.

Questions to Consider: Personal Habits

1. Is your loved one losing weight?
2. Is she sometimes showing signs of confusion?
3. Does she smell or look dirty?
4. Is her hair uncombed or unwashed?
5. Is clothing stained or smelly?
6. Has she had several falls, particularly falls resulting in breaks?
7. Is she too frail to do even basic vacuuming, bathing, and laundry independently?
8. Does she routinely get lost even going to familiar places?
9. Does she frequently forget names and words to the extent that it interferes with conversations?
10. Does she often lose things?
11. Does she forget to take medicine?
12. Does she forget whether or not she has taken medicine or does she sometimes take a second dose?
13. Does she forget to reorder medicines and run out?

As the senses dim, people may not notice odors or stains, but if they routinely wash themselves and their clothing, this is not a problem. If the person, bed, or clothing smells of urine or feces, it may be time to consider a move.

Certainly, everyone occasionally forgets a name or a word or loses something or forgets to take medicine once in a while-I'm only in my sixties and that happens to me sometimes. It may not be a problem if your mother once got locked out of the house or lost the keys or even had a stained bed from a bout of stomach flu. But if there is a consistent pattern of these occurrences, the situation needs to be addressed.

Signs of confusion should be taken very seriously. They can result from a variety of causes, all dangerous. Poor nutrition, dehydration, over-medication, a mini-stroke, or early dementia can all lead to confusion. It is crucial for a doctor to determine the cause of unusual or increasing confusion.

Problems with medicine are critical. Under or over dosing can cause serious health problems ranging from mild confusion to death.

The Kitchen

1. Is the refrigerator empty?
2. Does it contain spoiled or outdated food?
3. Are the pantry shelves empty?
4. Do they contain a balanced variety of foods?
5. Are dishes left piled up on the table or the sink?
6. Are trash containers overflowing?
7. Is a formerly neat kitchen cluttered?
8. Is the stove, toaster oven, or iron sometimes left on? If so, it is definitely time for a move.

For many seniors, the appetite dwindles, and they cannot count on bodily urges to tell them when they need to eat or drink. This is dangerous for many reasons. People who are undernourished or dehydrated may mimic symptoms of dementia such as confusion. They are also in greater danger of heat stroke. This lack of appetite coupled with difficulty shopping for food or preparing it, may cause seniors to eat poorly.

Canned foods and many frozen meals, while easy to prepare, are often very high in sodium, and thus are dangerous to people with high blood pressure. If the freezer is stocked with all frozen meals, the closets full of only cereal, bread, and canned soups, there is a good chance that the person is not getting the nutrition she needs.

Foods like tuna or even peanut butter are also easy to prepare, but contain some protein. Frozen vegetables contain needed vitamins and avoid the risk of waste or spoilage of fresh vegetables, or the high sodium content of canned products.

If food is left out and dishes left unwashed, there is an increased danger of bugs, rats, spoilage, and germs. So if nutrition and cleanliness in the kitchen become serious problems, it is time to get your loved one to move.

The Bathroom

1. Is there a grab bar in the tub or shower?
2. Are the bathroom floors dirty?
3. Are the toilets dirty?
4. Is the tub or shower dirty?
5. Is the hairdryer or shaver left plugged in or left on?
6. Are there wet or mildewed towels left out?
7. Does the laundry basket smell?

8. Are there stained or soiled clothes left in it for long periods of time?
9. Are toiletries like soap, shampoo, toilet paper, tissue, deodorant, toothpaste, powder etc. in the bathroom?
10. Do the towels look like they have been used?
11. Do they look like they have been washed recently?

The bathroom is the site of many accidents for the elderly. It is easier to walk into a shower than to climb in and out of a bathtub. Showers and tubs should have grab bars and seats. A hand-held shower head makes it possible for the frail elderly to sit while they shower. A long-handled scrubber makes it possible to wash the back or feet without twisting or bending, thus reducing the likelihood of a fall. A non-slip surface is essential in the tub.

A raised toilet with grab bars also makes the bathroom safer.

The House in General

1. Is the place cluttered?
2. Do newspapers and mail pile up unread?
3. Do bills go unpaid?
4. Is the door left unlocked?
5. Does she lock herself out regularly?
6. Are lights turned off at night?
7. Does she refuse to use heat or air conditioning when weather requires it because of the cost?
8. Are light bulbs replaced as needed?
9. Are there any obvious electrical problems that have not been repaired?
10. Are there any major plumbing problems that have not been fixed?
11. Is the house run down, in need of painting?
12. Is the lawn/garden maintained?
13. Are carpets worn, especially on steps?
14. Is the house in need of major work like roof or window replacement?
15. Do the walkway and steps get shoveled in snow?
16. Do floors need a good washing or vacuuming?

Clutter is a fire hazard as well as an accident waiting to happen for people with failing vision. A clear walking path is mandatory. Throw rugs and runners are a danger. They may slip or bunch, especially when someone is using a cane or walker on them.

Legal Options

It is often difficult to force a person to give up a license or move, especially if she is mentally competent. You can get help from the courts if you can prove that she is a danger to herself or others. But such action can result in a rift in the family just at the time that your loved one most needs your help. Court action should only be taken as a last resort and only when there is clear danger.

It might be better for your peace of mind for your family member to move, but it may be better for her peace of mind to stay in a beloved home. So make sure when you make the decision to try to get a person to move, it is because you truly believe that she is in danger staying alone. Your convenience or your peace of mind is not a good enough reason to encourage a move which is traumatic in the best of circumstances. And some perfectly rational people will say, "I have lived a good long life and I would rather stay in my house even knowing the dangers I face from a possible fall, than go to a nursing home and have a long, meaningless life." There is much to be said for this point of view. Most of us share it. At any rate, if you wish for a soul to soul relationship with your parent, you must listen closely to her wishes and concerns, rather than trying to impose your will "for her own good." Sometimes there are alternatives that can be tried to maximize safety in the house and allow the person to stay there longer while alleviating your worries.

Can She Still Drive?

---

* *Many aging drivers have slower response times.*
* *Drivers over 65 are twice as likely to die in car crashes as drivers 55-64.*
* *As drivers reach their 70's and 80's, those odds worsen.*
  (statistics from AAA Foundation for Traffic Safety)

Story: Car Trouble

Beth was an elegant, silver-haired lady, still beautiful in her late eighties. She swam daily, bowled weekly, and attended church faithfully. But one day she drove to the neighborhood supermarket, did her shopping, paid her bill, and went out to her car. She loaded the groceries into the trunk, climbed into the car, and froze. She absolutely could not remember what to do next. She asked a passing shopper for help. The shopper called the police who drove Beth to the hospital. It could have been a mini-stroke, but in her case it was the beginning of a very quick and very steep decline into dementia.

It is very difficult to get a parent to give up a license. In Beth's case, the hospital was required to file a report, and the state recalled her license. But in many cases the family is left to decide when a loved one is no longer fit to drive. Because visual and mental decline is often very slow, the person herself is very rarely able to recognize when she has declined to the point that she should not be driving.

Always discuss your concerns with her and offer her transportation options. If you think it is safe, compromise by asking her to only drive during the day, and only locally.

It is difficult to give up a car because it means losing independence. But, if your relative's vision or reflexes are such that she is not safe behind the wheel, and she will not give up the car, notify local police. It is better if the police tell her to stop driving than if you do. Think how terrible you and she will feel if she causes an accident in which she or others are injured when you knew that she should not have been driving.

Find out about local senior transport options or nearby public transportation. If possible, arrange for a driver one day a week, or find volunteers among her friends (or yours) to take her out once a week, so she won't feel stranded.

As we mentioned earlier, confusion can be a sign of many things. It can be the beginning of dementia, a sign of a physical illness, a sign of poor nutrition or hydration, or a sign of over or under medicating, among others. But a person experiencing confusion, regardless of the cause, should not be allowed to drive.

CHAPTER 2

Things to Do To Make the Home Safer

For a man's house is his castle, and one's home
is the safest refuge to everyone.
—Sir Edward Coke

Since most people are reluctant to leave home, there are many steps that can be taken to maximize the time your relative can stay at home. Put in an alarm system and get an alert necklace, which she can push if she is sick, hurt, or in danger.

Check on your loved one yourself or have neighbors or friends call or visit at least twice daily. If you cannot do it yourself, hire an aide to straighten up, do light shopping, laundry, and light cleaning at least twice a week. It would be good if that aide could stay in the house while your relative showers and washes her hair.

If your parent with early dementia lives with you or another adult, use an alarm system or a baby monitor to warn you if she wanders.

Most major religions have social service agencies that can help you find people to help you with personal care or house chores. In many cases fees are on a sliding scale based on one's ability to pay. Most cities also have agencies for the elderly that can help to provide these services. If you have very little time or live far from your loved one, it is possible to hire a geriatric case manager who will assess the needs and suggest necessary services to assist. Go to *www.caremanager.org* to find a qualified care manager near your parent. For other resources, check the annotated website list in the addenda.

Leave a list of emergency numbers in large print, by the phone. Leave a list of medicines to be taken daily and the times they are to be taken. If she is forgetful, or can't see well enough to tell one prescription bottle from another, put the meds in a separate little medicine box marked for each day of the week. Then if the box for that day is empty, she has taken the pills. For people who forget what day of the week it is, call in the morning. Say "Today is Monday June 1st. While I am waiting on the phone, take the pills in the box marked Monday."

Install grab bars around the toilet and in the bathtub. Put permanent, non-slip decals on the bathtub for better traction. If needed, put a plastic seat in the bathtub or bathroom so she can sit while washing.

Remove clutter on the floors. It is best to avoid area rugs, but if there are area rugs, make sure they have rubber backing, so they do not move when someone steps on them. Make sure carpet is not worn or frayed.

Find a pharmacy and food store that will deliver. If bills are left unpaid or she can't see well enough to do the checkbook, get an automatic bill-paying service or pay the bills yourself.

Make sure that things are where they belong, so people with limited vision can find them without falling over them.

Many seniors are only one fall away from needing assisted living or nursing care. Try to get your loved one to look at options with you before she needs them, so you will know what her preferences are if an emergency arises. This way you will not have the burden of looking and deciding on your own at the time of a crisis.

CHAPTER 3

Alternatives for Elder Living

Be nice to your kids. They will choose your nursing home.
—Bumper Sticker

There are many misconceptions about Americans warehousing their elderly parents, in nursing homes. In fact, less than 5% of seniors over age 65 live in nursing facilities. Only for frail elderly, those over 85, does the percentage in nursing homes become significant. It is important to realize that the children of frail elderly are themselves senior citizens, perhaps equipped to care for themselves, but rarely strong enough to deal with the needs of lifting, feeding, dressing, bathing, and perhaps diapering an elderly parent.

Depending on the physical and mental condition of the senior citizen, there are many options available besides nursing homes.

In some cases, it is possible for someone to **stay at home with an aide** or relative coming a few hours each day to shop, prepare meals or do light cleaning. For people needing a little help with bathing and dressing, it might be possible to have a part-time aide. If your parent had the foresight to purchase long term health care insurance, she may be able to get aides or nurses or therapy at home that will be covered by the insurance.

In San Francisco, residents at a city-run nursing home filed a lawsuit against the city claiming that disability rights laws allowed them to live at home and get care rather than living in a nursing home if the costs are the same or less than nursing home costs. In the past, city and state financial aid has only been available to those in nursing homes. It is too soon to know if other cities and states will agree to pay for homecare rather than forcing seniors into nursing homes to get financial aid.

The advantages of homecare are obvious. The cost to the city or state is significantly less for home health care as opposed to nursing home care. More importantly, the senior keeps most of her privacy and independence while staying in a place that is familiar to her. And she has friends and neighbors nearby. This option is available for people who are still fairly alert mentally, but perhaps frail physically. Unless an aide can stay all day every day, this option is not recommended for people with dementia or Alzheimer's who may turn on the stove and forget to turn it off, or forget to eat or take medicine when the aide is not there.

Most aides are honest, but they are also underpaid, so remove temptation. Remove valuables, and lock up cash, checkbooks, and credit cards. For more peace of mind, you might want to install video cameras in some rooms. This will help you to see how the aide treats your parent, and whether she works when you are not there to supervise.

A second option is **adult day care.** These programs provide supervision, age-appropriate activities, and meals. In some cases, they also provide transportation to and from the day care center. Find one that has supervised activities that allow people to use their skills such as sewing, cooking, gardening, or woodworking. Find a place that also has book discussions, crafts, and current events discussions, not one that is a glorified nursery school for adults. Adult day care is a good option for people with their faculties who do not wish to be home alone all day and for people with early stages of dementia. These places vary on whether they take severely impaired or incontinent people. If a place does take more severely impaired individuals, make sure there are separate rooms and activities for those without impairment. Having both groups in the same room is very depressing for intact individuals who are constantly being reminded by the presence of the dementia patients of what they already fear the most for themselves.

A less-expensive daytime option for those who are totally competent but lonely is a **senior citizen center**. Most communities have these now. They provide social activities, classes, trips, and sometimes meals for seniors. A few have transportation or arrange carpools for those who can't drive.

Another option is **moving in with family**. If the family's house is too small for her to have her own room without rearranging the sleeping arrangements for other family members, this decision may lead to tension in the family. If there is already anger or resentment between the aging parent and any other member of the family, having her move in will only exacerbate the problems. If there are problems in the family that don't relate to her, having her there may intensify those problems as well. Finally if all family members work or go to school, even if the family gets along well and wants her to come, she will be alone all day. Unless she is very independent or the family can find adult day care centers nearby or bring in an aide, this move will probably not be good for the aging parent who will be alone and lonely all day.

Since the baby-boomers have begun to age, there have been a plethora of **55 and older communities/ retirement communities** springing up around the country. These communities do not usually provide assistance. They are individual homes, condos, or apartments in a community where all or most of the residents are aging. The advantage to these places is that some have banks, doctors' offices, recreation facilities, a small restaurant or grocery, and a gym/pool on the grounds. Some, but not all, of these communities may have shuttle buses or maid service available (usually for an additional cost). These places are only for people who are physically and mentally capable of caring for themselves. Units are usually on one floor and multi-level condo buildings have elevators, so people do not have to climb steps. These are usually smaller and easier to care for than big homes. Many have laundry facilities in each home or condo unit. There is no supervisor or aide to check on a resident in a 55 and older community. This kind of place is inappropriate for someone with dementia or severe physical limitations. In most cases the resident must be responsible for her own care, laundry, cleaning, and meals.

Independent living facilities are another option. The resident has a private home or apartment, but there may be doctors, security, and maintenance people on call in emergencies. The residents still have their own kitchens and bathrooms, although many independent living facilities also offer the option of community dining for residents who don't want to cook. Facilities differ in the number of meals they provide.

One advantage is that there are many people the same age, and social activities are designed for the interests and abilities of older people. Another advantage is the privacy of a separate dwelling, coupled with the companionship of others in the community, and assistance in maintaining the house or providing meals. Many such facilities also offer transportation to shopping centers, supermarkets, and doctors' appointments. This option is better for people with mental competence. Aides and maid service are often available, but usually at an additional charge.

Usually staff will check on a resident who does not show up for meals. Residents are still expected to carry out most activities of daily living on their own. Some people may use walkers or even wheelchairs, but they must be able to take care of themselves. People who are very frail, need help dressing or bathing, or show signs of dementia should not be in independent living. No one will check to see that the stove is turned off or medicine is taken, so people who are forgetful would be a danger to themselves and others in such a facility.

In some parts of the country, **group homes** are available. In this setting, the aging parent has a private or semi-private room in a house that she shares with four or five other older residents. In some settings there is an aide who lives in or nearby as well. In other homes, the residents share the responsibility of cooking, cleaning, laundry. There are many advantages to this arrangement. First it is a house, not a nursing home, so it feels closer to the way the resident lived prior to moving. There is some level of independence, and the residents are still using some of their homemaking skills. There is companionship and help available. This living arrangement can be cheaper than maintaining a home alone. The disadvantage is shared bathrooms and shared common space. This arrangement may not offer enough supervision for people who are in serious physical or mental decline.

Assisted Living is an option that provides more care than retirement communities and less care than nursing homes. The resident has a private or semi-private room, meals and cleaning provided, assistance available for dressing or bathing, and medical assistance on the premises. The advantage is the resident can maintain some semblance of independence, while getting care and supervision needed. The disadvantage is that the aid provided is assistance. It is usually expected that the resident can carry out most of the activities of daily living independently. For example, aides may help a resident dress, but do not expect to have to completely dress the resident. Some Assisted Living facilities have showers in the bathroom in a resident's room, but many do not. They have a specially equipped bathroom in the hall and an aide will assist a resident at bath-time. In this case, residents bathe at the convenience of the aide, and they do not have complete privacy. In such places, a resident may be scheduled to bathe only two or three times a week. Many Assisted Living facilities will not take wheelchair-dependent residents, advanced Alzheimer's cases, or people needing toileting. Meals, transportation, and social activities are often available in Assisted Living facilities. The following are some questions to ask about an Assisted Living Facility. For a more complete list, see the list under nursing homes.

Assisted Living Evaluation

1. Are there choices at mealtime if the resident doesn't like the main meal? Will the kitchen staff accommodate special eating needs such as kosher, halal, vegetarian, sugar-free, low sodium, etc.?
2. How many meals are provided? Can visitors join the residents at meals? What is the charge for this?
3. Is there a beautician on the premises?
4. Is there a nurse on duty? What hours?
5. Is a doctor on site or on call?
6. Is there a chaplain? How many hours per week/month?
7. Do residents bathe themselves?
8. If not, how often are they bathed? Who determines when and how often a resident is bathed?
9. Is there a fire alarm and sprinkler system in every unit?
10. Are the units private or shared?
11. If shared, how do they determine who will share? Do they take into consideration common interests, common mental or physical state, or common bedtime schedules?
12. What is the ratio of aides to residents?
13. What training and security clearance do the aides have?
14. Are staff members required to get CPR and First Aid Certification?
15. What is the turnover rate among staff?
16. How many activities people are on at one time? What kinds of activities are provided?
17. Is there a transportation van? Where will it take residents?
18. Is there an additional charge for housekeeping, doing laundry, dispensing medications, or providing transportation?
19. Is there a gym, library, or swimming pool?
20. Is physical therapy available? How often? Is there an extra charge for it? Who decides if the resident will get therapy?

Continuing Care Communities

Story:

Mr. and Mrs. Jones bought into a beautiful apartment in the independent living portion of a continuing care community. The dining room was luxurious, the halls and public areas comparable to any good hotel.

But Mr. Jones died and Mrs. Jones developed dementia so she needed to move into the locked dementia unit. Because they had been high functioning when they moved in and the independent facilities were so lovely, they never bothered to look at the dementia unit. Furthermore, they felt it was too depressing to check out the assisted living or nursing home areas, so they didn't.

Mrs. Jones called the locked unit a dungeon. Her family agreed. The place had no sitting area, no programming, and blank dirty white walls. The huge financial buy-in to move into the facility guaranteed she could stay, but only in what the facility determined was the appropriate level of housing for her; however, it did not refund any money if she wanted to move to another facility. Therefore, she was trapped in the "dungeon" because she could not afford to go elsewhere if she didn't get back a portion of the initial buy-in.

Continuing Care Retirement Communities (CCRCs) run the gamut from independent living to nursing care in one community. These involve a substantial investment because the resident usually buys into the facility (an investment of $100,000 and up). Then there is a monthly fee that may be as low as $1000, but is often much higher. What the resident gets for her money is a condo or home while she is independent, and the guarantee that she can move to the assisted living and nursing facilities if she needs them in the future. People generally consider these when they are in fairly good health and can function on their own. They may be in the facility for ten or twenty years. Therefore, such a move must be made cautiously. When people check out such places, they shouldn't just look at the independent unit. They should check out the assisted living and nursing home and dementia unit facilities on the premises as well. Before signing a contract for such a place, the resident should have a lawyer review it.

Some questions to consider before moving into such a Continuing Care Community:

1. Is there an initial buy-in cost? How much is it?
2. What happens if a person moves in and doesn't like the place?
3. If the resident leaves, can she get any of the initial investment back?
4. Does the facility make any claims to ownership or control of the resident's property, income or estate?
5. When the resident dies, does the family get any of the initial investment back?
6. What is the financial situation of the parent company? You can check this at *www.standardandpoors.com*.

7. How will the investment be protected if the parent company goes bankrupt?

8. What are the monthly costs? Do they include meals, all activities, parking, and utilities? What services would bring an additional charge?

9. What guarantee is there that monthly costs won't escalate and become unaffordable? Is there a clause that limits how often or how much fees can be raised in a given year?

10. Is there a clause that guarantees the resident can stay if her money runs out?

11. Are there extra costs for transportation or is a free van available to take residents to appointments?

12. Is there an additional fee for parking or medicine distribution, or exercise facilities or classes?

13. Are there laundry facilities in each unit or each floor?

14. Is there an additional charge if a resident needs help with laundry or housekeeping?

15. Who decides when a resident moves out of independent living into assisted living or nursing care?

16. Is the facility approved by the Continuing Care Accreditation Commission? You can check this at *www.carf.org/aging*.

Nursing homes or Geriatric centers may be necessary for those who are physically or mentally impaired and need significant assistance in carrying out daily activities such as dressing, bathing, toileting, etc. When looking into a nursing home, check the qualifications of the staff.

Worksheet-Questions to Ask about Nursing Homes

Staff

1. What is the staff-resident ratio?
2. Does the home run a security check on its employees?
3. How many people does each aide assist?
4. What is the ratio of activities personnel to residents? If there are only one or two activities people on duty at a time, you can bet that most residents will not get to activities.
5. Are doctors or nurses always available?
6. Is there an on-site owner or manager?

7. How often are there staff meetings? How long are they? How many nurses, aides, and activities people are still available for the residents during these meetings?
8. What is the staff turnover rate?
9. What kinds of training/certifications are aides required to have?
10. Are staff members required to have CPR/ First Aid Certification?
11. Is there a staff chaplain? How many hours per week? What does the chaplain do? Are there regularly scheduled clergy visits, services, Bible study? Does the staff chaplain coordinate services for residents of other faiths?
12. Are there chaplains or religious volunteers from different faiths? How often? Do clergy from your religion come?

Activities

13. What activities are provided for the residents? Is there an additional cost for these activities?
14. Are there trips outside the facility? How often? How many residents can go? How is it determined who can go? What do these trips cost?
15. If the calendar says "music" does that mean outside entertainers or do the residents watch Lawrence Welk reruns or sit in a room with a radio on?
16. Are there supervised activities like gardening, art classes, carpentry, cooking, sewing that allow residents to use their skills?
17. Are there card games or game nights?
18. Are there physical activities such as walks, exercise classes, physical therapy? Do all residents participate? If not who determines which ones take part?
19. Are there mentally stimulating activities like book clubs, art programs, lectures, travel talks, current events, writing programs?
20. How often are outside people brought in for lectures or entertainment?

Rooms

21. How many people share a room?
22. Does the home attempt to match people with similar physical or mental abilities when determining room assignments?
23. What happens if roommates don't get along?
24. How big is the room?
25. What furniture is provided?

26. Can the resident bring her own furniture or furnishings to personalize the room?
27. Is there a lock box for valuables? Who has access to it?
28. How much storage space is there?
29. Is there wallpaper or paintings on the wall? Is the room physically attractive?
30. What is the physical layout of the room? Is there enough space for people to move about the room with a walker or wheelchair?
31. Can the resident personalize the room with pictures or a lamp or table of their own? Can residents have a clock, phone, television, radio, or calendar in the room?

Security

32. How is security? Who is in charge of security?
33. Are personal items likely to disappear?
34. What provision is there for securing valuables?
35. Can a resident's personal money be kept in a secure location? What arrangements are there for the resident to get access to her own money?
36. Are there wander guards on residents who might wander off?
37. Is there a buzzer access system to get into the building or to prevent confused residents from leaving?
38. Is there always someone at the front desk?
39. Do guests/workers have to sign in and out?

Meals

40. Are there alternate choices at meal-time if a resident doesn't like the main course of a meal? Is the alternative another hot entrée or a peanut butter sandwich?
41. Which meals are provided?
42. Do the residents all eat at one time or do they eat in shifts? What determines who eats in each shift?
43. Do all residents eat in the same room? If not, what determines which room a resident uses?
44. How does the staff identify residents with specific dietary restrictions? Do the residents wear color-coded bracelets to identify their special needs? (e.g. sugar free diets, food allergy restrictions, thickened liquids).

45. Do aides help those who cannot feed themselves? What is the ratio of aides or dining room workers to residents?
46. Does staff monitor to make sure all residents come to meals and to see how much a resident eats?
47. Do residents get assistance getting to the dining room?
48. Are meals provided in their room for ill residents?
49. How attractive is the dining room?
50. What is a typical menu for a week?

Finances

51. What does the place cost? Is there an initial entrance fee?
52. What is the monthly cost? What is included in that cost?
53. What is not included? (Is there an additional charge for laundry, medicine distribution, room cleaning, certain activities, transportation, etc.)
54. What guarantees are there that the resident can remain if she outlives her money?
55. What is the average yearly increase? Is there a maximum that rates can be raised from year to year?

Personal Hygiene

56. Are there private baths? If not, how often is a resident bathed and by whom?
57. Who helps with daily personal care such as sponge baths, brushing teeth, washing or combing hair, dressing and undressing?
58. Is there a barber shop/beauty shop on the premises? Is there an additional charge for these services? How much?
59. Who supervises to see that residents take baths, get hair washes, and change clothes enough to maintain cleanliness?
60. Can residents request aides of the same sex to provide personal services?
61. By what time of the day can residents expect to have been washed and dressed?
62. By what time can they expect to be prepared for bed?
63. Are residents routinely checked and treated for bedsores, skin irritation, dirty fingernails, long finger or toenails?
64. Are nail cutting and nail polishing services available? Is there an additional charge?

The Facility

65. Is there an enclosed garden area so residents can go outside without wandering off?
66. Is there a locked unit for Alzheimer's/dementia patients?
67. Is there a library?
68. Is there a kitchen or workshop that residents can use? (supervised). If yes, what protection is there to guarantee that residents cannot use the appliances unsupervised?
69. Are there one or more activity rooms large enough to accommodate most of the residents at one time?
70. Are there little lounges where residents can entertain guests?
71. How wide are the hallways? Are they usually cluttered with trashcans, med carts? Food carts? Are they wide enough for residents to pass by in wheelchairs even if there is a med cart or food cart in the hallway?
72. Are the doors alarmed or code-activated so residents with wander-guards cannot get out?
73. Are nurses stations arranged so nurses can see into the rooms or at least see the help-needed light outside each room?
74. Are there emergency pull cords in each room and each bathroom?
75. Is there a separate room for the beautician?
76. Is there a separate room for physical therapy? For occupational therapy? How well-equipped are these rooms for the kinds of help your parent needs?
77. Are they staffed by licensed physical therapists or therapy assistants or aides?
78. How often can a family member get therapy?
79. Who decides if therapy is needed?
80. Who decides when the therapy will end?

Emergency Situations

1. If it is a multiple-floor facility, is there more than one elevator?
2. What arrangements are there to get residents to and from their rooms during a power outage when the elevators can't be used?
3. What are the emergency evacuation plans in case of flood or fire? How often are there drills to practice them?
4. What is the normal procedure for a medical emergency?
5. What is the normal response time when someone rings the emergency bell in their room?

CHAPTER 4

Making the Move

We have been moved already beyond endurance, and need rest.
—John Maynard Keynes

As much as possible, the senior should be involved in the decision-making process about her move. She is the one who will have to live with the conditions in the new place. Expect anger and depression at first even if she made the move willingly. There is also the possibility that she will experience some confusion after the move. This confusion, which also often occurs during hospital stays or after accidents, may or may not be temporary.

Aging is a series of losses, all of which need to be mourned. First it is loss of health or strength or physical abilities. Then it may be loss of memories, mental abilities, loved ones. Moving from an independent setting to a nursing home is a profound loss—of privacy, of freedom, of personal property, of independence, of choices. Imagine moving from a home or apartment where you lived alone to a relatively small room, which you will share with a total stranger who you may not like or trust. Imagine leaving the place where your children grew, where you knew the neighbors, where your spouse died, where you chose the furniture and pictures in every room. You left behind gifts, books, jewelry, photos with sentimental values and beautiful memories attached to them to a place where you have a bed, a closet and a bureau-not of your taste or choice. Maybe the resident can hang a few of her favorite pictures, but certainly it isn't wise to bring much of value with her. But the loss of the physical things doesn't compare to the loss of privacy.

Sharing a room and a bathroom with a stranger may be great fun in a college dorm when it is done by choice, but it is quite another experience when it is done after years of independent living as an acknowledgment that a person is no longer physically or mentally able to care for herself.

Imagine being an adult suddenly being told when to go to bed, when to get up, what to eat, when to bathe. Imagine needing the aid of total strangers to help you dress and bathe. Think of the loss of self-respect involved with incontinence, when strangers must put a diaper on you, and they change it at their convenience, not yours. This may be especially traumatic for older women when the staff member doing the dressing and toileting is male. The losses involved in moving into a nursing home are profound. They are real, and the depression these losses sometimes engender is also real. If you can talk about the losses and acknowledge them, perhaps the adjustment will be easier. You, as the child, may also feel guilty for having done this to your mother, and this will be made worse if she is constantly berating you for abandoning her. Whenever possible, give her some choice in choosing a facility. For many seniors, it is not the facility per se, but the sense that her life is no longer in her control, that leads to depression. Try to return some control to her in deciding on the facility, choosing how to decorate her room, deciding which items to take or leave behind. When a parent is constantly angry at you for the choices you made, it is hard for you not to allow the guilt to eat away at you. Try never to make a promise you may not be able to keep. (e.g. Rather than saying, "I will never put you in a nursing home," say "I will care for you as long as I am able.")

Remind yourself (and your mother) often that you must maintain your health so you can continue to provide for her. Remind yourself that having her live at home with you could be emotionally and physically draining on you and your family. It can jeopardize the mental and physical health of your family and strain your marriage and family relationships. Furthermore, if you work or travel, your mom would be alone which is not good for her if she is physically or mentally impaired.

Listen to her hurt and anger about moving from her home and acknowledge her feelings. But also tell her the reasons you think the move will benefit her.

So what can you do to ease the adjustment to a nursing home? Bring pictures, photographs, or plants to personalize the room. Make sure the room has a clock and a calendar. One day is pretty much the same as another in a nursing facility, but a calendar with special days or events marked on it, gives the resident something to look forward to. Find out what activities are available and try to get your mother involved in some of them.

CHAPTER 5

Visiting

I was sick and ye visited me.
—Matthew 25:35

Visit often and if possible provide a telephone in the room so your mother still has contact with the outside world. Bring cards or Mah Jong games, or chess with you. If your mother likes music, bring a tape recording of her favorite songs. Try to focus conversations on people you know or current events, so she will not be focusing only on the nursing home life all of the time.

The worst part of living in a nursing home is feeling useless. This is a "doing" oriented society and many in nursing homes feel that when they can no longer "do" they have no right to be. It can be helpful to find things that mom can still do that will show her that she is still useful and needed. She might crochet or knit something for an upcoming wedding or birth in the family. She might put together a family tree or record her memories to provide a living history for her grandchildren. She might call a friend who is a shut-in or attend services daily if the nursing home provides them. If she is good at crocheting or art or writing, she might even organize a workshop in the nursing home to teach others.

But it is equally important to stress the value of being. We are not after all human doings, but human beings. We need to see the frail as human beings containing a divine soul, and we need to encourage them to see themselves that way, regardless of their limitations. Many elderly, even those who were not religious in younger years, may look for spirituality in later years. After all, they are coming to the end of their lives and they know it, so they might want some confirmation on the value of the life they've led and even some speculation of what comes next. Therefore, it is good to find a nursing home that encourages chaplaincy visits and religious observances.

Many family members have difficulty visiting nursing homes. In some cases it is fear of their own mortality that makes visiting difficult. However, old age is not contagious, and if being in such a place does engender fears that you may end up this way yourself some day, wouldn't it be better to end up that way with visitors than without them? Some people don't go because they don't know what to do or say. That is the mistake of the "human doing" syndrome. It is okay to just be there without doing anything. This is called the ministry of presence and it is the hardest thing to learn. We want to be able to fix things, to do something, to say something, but sometimes all the seniors need is someone to be there, to hold their hand, to listen if they want to speak. And we don't have to listen necessarily to fix things; some things are unfixable, but we can listen to validate their feelings about those things we can't fix.

It is hardest to visit the relatives who stir up guilt every time you come. The answer is not to stop visiting, but to establish rules for the visit. Let your mother know that you want to visit and you will visit, but you will leave if she starts a harangue-then do it! Try to talk about topics of interest to her, or bring music, or photos or games she likes and enjoy them together. But when she starts the criticism or guilt talk, tell her you will not stay for this, but you love her and she will visit again. Remind yourself that some parents will never be pleased and nothing you do will be good enough to suit them. In that case, do the best you can do under the circumstances, so that you are at peace with yourself. Don't let your parent or the nursing staff intimidate or guilt you into doing more than you want to do. This is especially true when you are caring for a parent who did not care for you.

However, if your mother has complaints about the treatment at the home, take her seriously. It is possible her complaints are meant to create guilt or are the result of paranoia, but it is also possible that there is neglect or even abuse. Does she have unexplained bruises? Does she complain about all the caregivers or only one? Speak to other residents or other family members and see if they have the same complaints. Try to visit at different times of the day, especially at first, to see what time the staff gets her out of bed in the morning, and whether they take her to the bathroom or change her regularly. Have meals with her a few times to see if her complaints about food are justified. And be aware that even in the nicest nursing homes, the residents that have regular visitors will get the best treatment by the staff. Most nursing homes are chronically short-staffed, and they don't always get to everyone in a timely fashion. But they want to give the appearance of efficiency to families, so the staff will take better care of those who have frequent visitors. Chronically demanding or nasty residents or family members will antagonize the staff which may result in less care for the resident. But if there are unexplained bruises, file a report and ask to contact an ombudsman. Every county or state has an ombudsman to mediate problems with abuse or nursing home care issues. Good nursing homes have signs posted around the facility with information about contacting the ombudsman. If you are not satisfied with the facility's handling of a complaint, ask them how to contact the ombudsman. If they refuse to give you this information, call your state Department of Aging.

Remember that the staff is only human. Just as you wish to avoid visits if your mother is constantly angry or demanding, the staff will also try to avoid the residents who are most unappreciative and demanding. It is very helpful to make the nursing home resident aware that her own treatment of the staff may very well affect their treatment of her. This can be a problem with residents in various stages of dementia who may scream, curse or use ethnic slurs. Even though the resident cannot control the outbursts, they can nevertheless be hurtful to the staff. Do what you can to be extra considerate to staff members who may be taking abuse from your loved one.

To make the stay as pleasant as possible for your mother, try to have family get-togethers especially for holidays, which include her. If she is too frail to leave the facility, then bring some family gatherings to the nursing home.

Finally, be kind to yourself. You are doing the best that you can in a very difficult situation.

When your confused mother says, "I want to go home" don't say "This is your home" or "You can't go home anymore." You could say, "You need to stay until your memory improves or until you get better (even though you know that won't happen.) Try deflecting the request by saying, "Lunch is coming soon" or "There is Bingo this afternoon. Why don't you stay for that?"

For people who are mentally alert, but physically frail tell them what they need to be able to do physically to be able to live independently. For example, "When you can get out of bed, transport yourself to the bathroom, cook your meals, we can talk about having you go home."

Summary of Visiting Strategies

All our interior world is reality-and that perhaps more so than our apparent world. Marc Chagall as cited in **Caring for**

Your Parents, (Delehanty, Ginzler, p. 115.)

1. Your aging parent may often retreat to her "interior world." You may get insights into her feelings or learn wonderful stories about her childhood if you join her there instead of trying to pull her back into your world.

2. Treat her as an adult. Do not speak about her in her presence as if she isn't there. Don't speak to her as if she is the child and you are the parent. She is the parent and she deserves the respect of being treated as such.

3. Use simple instructions—one step at a time—when you want her to do something. But work at avoiding the condescending or exasperated tone that can so easily creep in.

4. Respond to her feelings. Learn to pay attention to facial expression, and body language, especially when she can't communicate verbally.

5. Be flexible. You may have come in with a particular agenda for the day, but she may not be physically or emotionally equipped that day to do what you had in mind. Find out what she wants to do, even if it's looking through the same photo album she looked through on the last ten visits. You remember that you did it before, but if she has short term memory loss, she doesn't. So looking at the album for the tenth time gives her as much pleasure as if she were seeing it for the first time.

6. Give encouragement.

7. Be patient. She isn't deliberately taking twenty minutes in the bathroom when you visit. It just takes longer to do everything when you are older and frailer, and her concept of time isn't the same as yours.

8. Don't scold. (That is another example of treating the parent as child).

9. Talk to her as if she understands; even people with dementia have moments of lucidity, so sometimes she does understand.

10. Approach from the front. This way you will avoid startling her.

11. Always identify who you are and who any guests with you are. Do not ask, "Do you remember me, or do you know who this is?" It is embarrassing to her when she doesn't know, but thinks that she should know, who someone is.

12. Give hugs and gentle touch. Thin skin can be very sensitive, so take your clues about touching from her response to it. If she seems amenable to touch, you could do things like putting lotion on dry skin or manicuring her nails, or fixing up her hair. Physical contact has been shown to be an important element for mental health, and people in nursing homes rarely get enough gentle contact.

13. Establish eye contact, sit near her, and always talk directly to her. Don't cover your mouth when you talk. If her hearing is failing, she needs the visual cues of your mouth position and facial expression to help her understand you. If she has hearing problems, you may speak slightly louder, but don't shout. Sometimes hand gestures will help communication.

14. To encourage conversation, use open-ended questions that require more than a yes/no answer.

15. Create outlets for her physical tension. People with Alzheimer's are often very restless. They need to move. Did she used to enjoy dancing? Bring a tape and dance with her. Suggest taking a walk, particularly if the facility has outdoor gardens.

16. Never argue or rationalize.

17. Sing familiar songs, tunes, hymns. Bring tapes especially of her favorite kinds of music.

18. If the visit starts to get bad because she becomes hostile or agitated, tell her you are leaving; then go. If you wish, return a short time later to see if the bad mood has passed. If it hasn't, tell her when you expect to see her again, and leave.

19. Bring her favorite snacks or goodies to eat and drink together, but always be mindful, however, of her dietary restrictions and mealtimes.

CHAPTER 6

Caring for Yourself

If I am not for myself, who is for me? And if I am only for myself,
what am I? And if not now, when?
—Hillel in **Ethics of the Fathers I.14**

Care-giving Facts

1. 20% of caregivers suffer from depression
2. 44 million Americans are caregivers for spouse, parent, or other adult
3. 25% juggle work and care-giving responsibilities
4. 50% of caregivers have childcare and eldercare obligations
5. 20% of caregivers leave their job or cut back their work hours
6. 40% of families suffer financial hardship as a result of paying for care
7. 31% lose all family savings due to costs of care
8. Caregivers are more likely to have chronic health problems than non-caregivers the same age

Sometimes you may feel like a rubber band being stretched at one end by the demands of your job, children, and grandchildren, and at the other end by the needs of your aging parent or spouse. But remember, when rubber bands are stretched too far, they break. To protect yourself, learn the most important word in the English language-NO! Children learn it as one of their very first words, so why do we adults, particularly female adults, have such a hard time using it? Women are trained to be caregivers, and we feel guilty when we can't care for those we love. Set realistic expectations for yourself. You can't do it all! Ask for help from family, friends, religious community, and public sources. Make time for the things that give your joy. If seeing your grandchildren makes you happy, give yourself time to do it. But say NO to babysitting jobs that wear you out.

In your free time, surround yourself with upbeat people and avoid those who bring you down. Locate respite care facilities, adult day care, family or friends, local or religious volunteer groups that can give you a break.

Figure out what is the best stress release for you: a day at the spa or the beauty parlor, an hour in the gym or the pool, a luncheon date with friends. Then do it! Stress weakens the immune system. If you do not care for yourself, you will get sick, at which point you are no good to anyone. My stress release is an hour in the morning to swim or line dance. I schedule that time for myself before I schedule business appointments, babysitting for my grandkids, or shopping for my mother. I tell my mother when to make her doctors' appointments so they do not interfere with my time. Occasionally a doctor's appointment must be scheduled on my time; but then I plan a different treat for myself later in the day, perhaps a lunch out with friends.—Carol

My stress release is quiet time in the evening to read or bake or embroider. It gives me time to unwind from the stresses of the day.-Joan

Find the time and the stress release that works for you. If you don't get time for yourself, you may become angry at the person you are caring for. Resentment isn't good for you or for your relationship with your parent. Except in true emergencies, do not sacrifice your special time.

The pressures of care-giving are only amplified if you are working, because there are only so many hours in a day after work to do your own chores, do your mother's errands, visit grandchildren, spend time with your spouse, and give yourself time for what you need. But don't make satisfying your needs the thing that is sacrificed due to time limitations. The dust will still be there next week if you don't get to it today. If finances allow, maybe you can hire a part-time housekeeper or cook or shopper to pick up the slack if you don't have a spouse, friends, or other family who are willing to pitch in.

If it is possible, hire a care manager or an aide to do the errands for your parent if you decide to take a vacation. If the chance to take a vacation comes, grab it, but get trip insurance if you or your parents have real health issues.

Listen to calming music in your car on the way to a visit. If needed, stop and do a breathing meditation to calm and slow yourself down before you go inside. (See the list of Psalms and inspirational readings, including a breathing meditation at the end of this book.)

CDs like Barbara Streisand's **Higher Ground**, or **Infinite Oceans**(classical music with ocean sound in the background are relaxing. Reading poetry, Psalms or healing books such as **Reflections: Readings Of Spirituality, Gratitude and Love** can also slow you down and relax you before making a nursing home visit. For those who can do meditation, I highly recommend it. Bernie Siegel's **Guided Imagery and Meditation** is great for beginning meditation. Find a peaceful place or a spot of great natural beauty and just sit there and breathe quietly for five minutes. If you don't have time to take a yoga or Tai Chi class, give yourself just 5-10 minutes to do your favorite exercises from the class. We can absolutely guarantee from personal experience that if you don't give yourself this time when you are under stress, your body will break down physically and force you to take a break. Isn't it better to take the time off on your own terms than to do it because you have shingles, pneumonia or the flu?

Warning signs of caregiver burnout

1. Depression
2. Apathy
3. Resentment
4. Sleeplessness or constant sleeping
5. Fatigue
6. Recurring physical ailments
7. Loss of appetite or binge-eating
8. Feeling stressed
9. Mood swings/irritability
10. Increased use of medications/alcohol
11. Social withdrawal

(This list is adapted from the August 2007 AARP DVD: **Caring for Those You Care About**). To find out how to obtain a copy, e-mail *caregiving@aarp.org*

Long Distance Caregivers

It is particularly difficult to be a child living in another part of the country (or the world), when your parent needs help. Before you make the journey to take care of your parent's problems, gather as much information as you can.

If at all financially possible, hire a geriatric care manager to coordinate all of the components of care necessary. Check *www.caremanager.org* to find qualified people in your parent's area.

1. Determine what type of help is needed: wound care, physical therapy, legal advice, medical appointments, personal care, housekeeping, housing changes, transportation etc.
2. Gather information on line about housing options, geriatric care managers, eldercare lawyers, gerontologists (eldercare doctors), or state services in your parent's state. Most states have a department on aging that can direct you to their resources. E.g.: In Pennsylvania go to *www.aging.state.pa.us* or *www.longtermcare.state.pa.us* for information.
3. Identify key people you can count on: family, friends, neighbors, clergy or religious agencies, elder-transport services, senior centers, homecare agencies, geriatric care managers. Get a list of their names, addresses, and phone numbers.
4. Figure out which issues can be handled by phone or e-mail and which ones require your presence. Do as much as you can by phone or e-mail before you schedule a visit.
5. Make all appointments before you schedule your trip.
6. When you visit, you must cover all the business, but schedule some social time for you and your parent as well.

PART II

Scenes from Nursing Homes

People with Alzheimer's may have trouble with mental processes, may have
trouble finding the words to express the meaning in their heads,
but their feelings are intact. They still bleed. They feel pain, embarrassment,
joy, humor, other people's interest in them, companionship,
loneliness, boredom. They can feel useful and they can feel useless.
Reprinted with permission by New Harbinger Publications, Inc.
Talking to Alzheimer's, Claudia Strauss
www.newharbinger.com

The following vignettes, sometimes poignant, sometimes sad, sometimes humorous, express the humanity and the feelings of these residents. They are presented with respect and love as expressions of the interests, the needs, the feelings of these seniors. Each vignette is followed by suggestions for developing meaningful interaction in similar situations.

Dealing With Death

The Widow Who Didn't Know

Sharon was in the middle stages of Alzheimer's. She was wheelchair-bound. She needed more care than her aging husband could give her, so she moved into a nursing home. Still, she seemed quite alert at times. She regularly participated in religious services. She took part in many other activities as well. Her husband visited nearly every day.

When her husband died suddenly, her children decided it would be too much for Sharon to handle, so they didn't tell her.

Ten days later, I was leading services, and Sharon was there as usual. When the services ended and the other residents left, I found Sharon sitting in a corner sobbing as if her heart would break.

I went over to her, and she was embarrassed by her crying. "I shouldn't feel like this. This isn't like me. I shouldn't be crying like this," she said. "I'm so sad. I just can't stop crying. I don't know what to do." I asked her why she was so sad, and she replied, "I don't know, but I'm just so sad." I sat with her; I held her hand. I told her she had a right to her feelings and a right to cry if she felt sad. We talked for a while and she mentioned her children. I asked her if she had told them that she was feeling sad. She replied, "No my children don't like to talk to me about sad things."

The incident upset both Joan and me profoundly. We understood that the children were trying to protect Sharon from pain and sadness. But they hadn't done that. She knew something was wrong, and she was sad. She sensed that her children were keeping something from her. She still felt the pain and sadness, but she couldn't verbalize the reason. She didn't think she had the right to feel sad and to cry, and she didn't know what to do with her feelings. If her family had told her the truth, she would have still felt sad, but she would have known why. She would have had friends and family and staff with whom she could have discussed her loss and to whom she could turn for comfort. She would have known what to do with her grief and we would have known what to do for her. But having been ordered by the family not to tell her, the staff was limited in the help they could offer her. Under other circumstances I could have said mourner's prayers with her and held a memorial service for her husband. She would have had a service to attend, family, friends and staff to support her, and prayers to say. But the big secret deprived her of this comfort.

Suggestions for Interaction

Even people with severe Alzheimer's seem to sense when something is wrong or someone is missing. Even when they can't identify the loss, reactions such as crying or extreme agitation will often occur.

I understand that families want to protect their loved ones, but in this case and others like it, the loved one is not protected from the feelings, only from understanding them.

Those who are not able to deal with loss will usually suppress it. I have seen people with dementia simply forget that their beloved spouse is dead if they are not able to deal with the loss. So my gut reaction in situations like this is to encourage family members to tell nursing home residents of a loss. Your family should have support from social workers or clergy when you tell your parent. Then she could even attend the funeral, or at least have a memorial service at the nursing home. She can light candles (electric if fire codes don't permit real candles), say prayers, and observe traditional mourning processes.

If she then forgets that her husband is dead, it is a judgment call for the family and staff to decide whether to remind her of the death, bearing in mind that when she is told, she will experience the initial sense of loss all over again. Sometimes one can acknowledge the feeling of loss without reminding your loved one of the death. "You really miss him right now, don't you?" You can encourage her to reminisce about the absent spouse, or look at photos, if that is helpful rather than upsetting.

Death and Money

Story: Is the Money Mine?

Mrs. Cohen was asking for her husband. My friend gently reminded Mrs. Cohen of the funeral she had attended and the prayers she had said earlier in the week. Mrs. Cohen said, "He's dead?"

"Yes," my friend replied sympathetically.

Then Mrs. Cohen continued, "Does that mean all the money belongs to me now?"

Never presume to know what someone is feeling after the death of a spouse. If the relationship was a bad one, the spouse may feel relief, not grief. Even if the relationship was a good one, the person may be feeling anger or a sense of abandonment rather than grief. By listening carefully, you can find out what she feels, rather than projecting what you would feel in a similar situation. Even if the relationship was a poor one, even if the deceased was cruel, abusive, unfaithful, or neglectful, the survivor may feel sad. The survivor may be mourning the loss of the person or the loss of the opportunity to mend the relationship. Some people mourn what they had and lost; some mourn what they had and didn't appreciate; some mourn what they never had, should have had, and now never will have. Only by listening carefully to the survivor can you help her deal with whichever loss she is facing.

The Power of Love

Story: Isn't She Beautiful

Bella sat bent over in her wheelchair, her body twisted from the ravages of arthritis, Parkinson's, and a stroke. People walked past her in the hall, ignoring her. She was just one more old broken body in a nursing home full of them.

Finally a nurse saw her there and wheeled her into the room of her husband of 50 years. He smiled as she came into the room and he said to the nurse, "Isn't she beautiful?" Bella's face lit up at the sound of his voice, and I realized it was true. She was beautiful.

Older people, like all people, need to feel noticed, loved and appreciated. Residents who are severely confused or even comatose often react to the voice of a loved one. People who don't visit "because she won't even know I am there" are wrong. Tests of breathing patterns, heart beat etc. show that even a comatose person's body may react to a loved one's voice even if the reaction is not verbal or overt.

Suggestions for Interaction

Visit! Talk to the person even if she can't talk to you. Tell her about current events, the family, sports, travel, books or other things that interested her when she was well. Bring photos to show or music to listen to together. Massage or put lotion on her hands or feet if she isn't sensitive to touch.

The Power of Social Interaction

A Game of Gin Rummy

I walked into the group home where Rita lived. It felt more like a home than an institution. Four other women lived there, all in various stages of Alzheimer's. I'd known Rita for 30 years, but although she was as sweet as always, it was clear she didn't know who I was. When someone suggested a game of gin rummy, I was skeptical. She didn't remember old friends; she didn't remember what she had eaten an hour ago. How would she remember the rules to a complicated game? But we played—and she won all three games! And I realized two things. We had met on common ground, and that ground was holy. And in those moments when she played and won, she was whole and she was happy.

Suggestions for Interaction

Bring a book, a magazine, a newspaper. People retain their ability to read well into Alzheimer's. They may reread the same story twenty times as if each time is the first, but they get pleasure out of the reading each time. You may want to talk about the story or let them tell you about it.

If the person was an avid game or card player, try to play a favorite game with them. If you sense confusion, you can always stop. But many times people are able to play games they learned when they were young even though they may not be able to learn a new game or hobby.

The same is true of skills like sewing, knitting, quilting, painting, or doing puzzles. The time may come when they can no longer do these things, but many retain those abilities much longer than you might think. So if you share a hobby like knitting or sewing with the person you are visiting, bring supplies and do a craft together. When the time comes that she can no longer knit, she might still enjoy holding the wool for you as you knit. Just the feel of a familiar texture can sometimes give pleasure.

The Power of Prayer

Good Shabbas

Dr. Fishman came to services every week. He was in a geri-chair, in the end stages of Alzheimer's. I'd never heard him speak. But still he came, accompanied by his lady friend Tonya. She was of a different faith, but she came with him every week to turn the pages of the prayer book for him, to pat his hand, to help him with the juice served at the end of the service. Once when we were alone, Tonya talked to me about how bright Dr. Fishman had been, how interesting he had been to talk to, how much she missed that communication.

At the end of one service, I went around as usual shaking hands and greeting everyone. When I got to Dr. Fishman, I said, "Good Shabbas." Tonya and I looked at each other in amazement as he clearly replied, "Good Shabbas" and then immediately lapsed back into silence.

I never heard him speak again, and only a few weeks later he died, with Tonya by his side. But I often think of Dr. Fishman. I never question now whether what I do matters. Even if it was only once, even if it was only for a second, prayer got past a broken body, past a broken mind, and touched a living soul.

Since the experience with Dr. Fishman, I have had others like it. Prayer, especially when sung, has a way of reaching through the outer damaged body to find the intact soul. I know this. I have seen it. I have seen a woman who doesn't know where she is, perhaps not even who she is, hear the words to a prayer. She taps into some memory from her distant past and begins to sing along with me. It gives me goosebumps. The moment is holy.

There are times when I sing a prayer "Peace To You" at the start of services in a nursing home, and my congregants join in. It is a cacophony of sound that would make a music teacher cringe. But it touches my soul. It is the moment for me when the Sabbath really arrives. And there are times when I would swear I can feel God's spirit in the room with us.

Story: Hannah at Church

Hannah was a Jewish lady who had a private room. She didn't visit much with the other residents. She was happy to sit in her room. She delighted in the Public Address system which she thought was a new kind of phone that came through the ceiling. Every time announcements were made, she would answer them. One Sunday, the staff was surprised to see Hannah come to church. After the service, she approached an Activity Staff person. "You know I am Jewish, but I always wanted to go to a Christian church service."

The staff member asked, "Well, what did you think of the service?"

Hannah replied, "Boy, you sure took a lot from us!"

Doris and the three faiths

Doris was a very spiritual lady. She attended all religious services at the facility where she lived. She'd go to the Catholic service on Sunday morning, the Protestant services Sunday afternoon, and the Jewish services on Friday evening. She knew all the prayers, the order of the services, and all the appropriate music. She let each of the respective clergy think that she was a member of their congregation. When she passed away, she had three memorial services.

Jane and the Christmas tree

Jane was a very spirited and spiritual lady. She had been a teacher most of her life. Jane just loved Christmas, and most of all, she loved Christmas trees. She was always ready to help put up and decorate the trees in her nursing home. And every evening after supper during the holiday season, Jane would disassemble one of the trees. She would take the ornaments off and stash them in a dresser drawer. And every morning after breakfast, Jane and an activity staff member would redecorate the tree.

All of these stories have a common theme. Faith is extraordinarily important to the aging, even those who were not religious in their earlier years. They are coming to the end, and they know it. Faith makes the last years easier. Older residents seem to be more tolerant of different faiths. Spiritual connection is more imperative to them, and they are willing to get it wherever and however they can.

Suggestions for Interaction

Bring Bibles, books of psalms or spiritual readings to read together. Arranging a clergy visit is also important. You can bring a CD or tape or DVD of a service or religious songs. Sing with your parent, read psalms, tell Bible stories together. If possible, take her out to services.

The Power of Care-giving

Tammy

Suzie had Tammy, a white stuffed pussycat. Suzie clutched Tammy to her heart. Over the dozen years she lived at the facility, a dozen "Tammys" were loved to disintegration. Suzie knew that Tammy wasn't real. But she had once owned a white cat, and she liked to pretend that the stuffed animal was her old cat.

The Baby

Anh Lee was an Asian woman. Her English wasn't very good, and it must have been difficult for her because she rarely had people who could talk with her. But wherever she went, she had a doll on her lap. She rocked it, she cuddled it, and she sang to it. That "baby" gave her a purpose and she was content as long as she had her "baby" to tend.

People need physical contact, and residents in nursing homes rarely get affectionate touch. Those stuffed animals provided a gentle touch and gave the residents that much needed physical contact. In addition, all people need to feel useful. Caring for those animals and dolls gave the residents a sense of purpose.

For this reason, many nursing homes provide stuffed animals or real animals for the residents to hold and care for. More homes now have visiting or live-in pets. The residents love to hold these animals and care for them. It provides touch and purpose. For women this taps into the care-giving skills that were a crucial part of their earlier life.

Petey

May had real problems with coming to live in a nursing home. She was verbally abusive to the staff. At one point she threatened to escape by throwing a trashcan through a window. But then one day, May won Petey at Bingo. Petey was a life-size stuffed dog with pointed ears and a handkerchief around his neck. May loved Petey. She took him for walks, fed him, and even got other residents to watch him for her. Then she decided she should get a paycheck so she could take better care of Petey. Every day, May got a "check" from the business office for looking after her "dog."

May's story is an example of the power of care-giving. It also leads directly into the new section: the power of feeling financially independent.

The Power of Financial Independence

It's surprising how often the issue of money comes up in conversations with residents. Most parents of Baby Boomers survived the depression. They grew up in the "work hard, and save your money" generation. It is hard to overestimate how important that sense of financial security is to them. That is reflected in the story of May who liked getting her "check" to care for Petey. It is reiterated in the following stories as well.

Harry's Dollar

When Harry came to the dining room, he refused to eat. "I don't have the money to buy lunch." The aide tried to explain that his insurance covered his meals, but Harry still refused to eat. Finally, the aide handed him a dollar out of her own pocket. "This is yours. When I bring you your lunch, you can pay me with this." Harry agreed. When the aide brought the lunch, she asked Harry for the dollar in payment. "Oh, no," said Harry. "You told me insurance paid for my lunch. So I'll just keep this dollar."

The Donkey

Millie came to Bingo and won a stuffed donkey. Millie kept a close eye on her donkey until several months went by. Then one day, she announced that she wanted to sell him. Jokingly, a staff member asked for a commission for helping to sell the donkey.

Millie said, "Nothing doing! I've fed and cared for this donkey for months and fattened him up too. I deserve all the money!"

Suggestions for Interacting

When your parent expresses concern about money or about how her bills are being paid, don't reply "Don't worry. I'm taking care of it." Tell her "Insurance covers it" or "Medicare covers it." Tell her that she worked all her (or her husband worked all his life) so she would have those protections that are paying the bills. Make it clear that this is not charity, and that she earned the benefits she is now receiving. She doesn't want to think that you are paying her bills. She comes from the generation that did without for themselves so they could leave a legacy to their children. If she has stock investments or CD's that give interest, tell her she has income from that to pay her bills. Having lived through the depression she is naturally afraid of being without sufficient funds. She is equally afraid of being a financial burden on you. Make it clear that meals and hair appointments are paid for by insurance or billed to her accounts.

It is never a good idea to leave large amounts of money in a nursing home, but if it makes her feel secure to have a dollar in her pocket, let her have it.

The Power of Feeling Useful

Brian's List

Brian had early onset dementia. He was admitted to a nursing home at age 58. He wandered through the halls. He would only talk to residents and staff he liked. One day he came into the Activity Room and sat at the director's desk where a pen and paper were set out. He proceeded to write the numbers 1-20 in sequence down the left side of the paper. He did this constantly for several weeks until one day he wrote the following:

1. Everybody is here for an interview.
2. Time to leave.
3. Get a bicycle and ride home.
4. I'd like to go on a picnic.
5. Take 5 minutes and heal your heart.

It's possible that list-making made him feel useful. It may very well have been something he did in business. More importantly, this writing became his way to communicate with staff and family. It provided an outline that family and staff could use to get him to communicate about things that were important to him. They would talk to him and he would write his answer. His writing gave insight into his feelings. They became his way "to heal his heart." The things that he wrote gave insight into the kind of person he was, and what he liked to do before he came to the facility.

Anna

Anna was in the early stages of dementia, and she was often confused. But like must Alzheimer's or dementia sufferers, she had moments of amazing lucidity. For example, one time she said to a staff member, "You people forget that I'm not in my right mind. But I want to be helpful. Just tell me what you want me to do, and I'll do it."

This story shows two important points. Residents in the early stages of dementia are often aware that they are confused. And they still want to be useful.

My Farm

Harvey spent all day every day sitting and staring out a glass door. His view was of an open field beyond which was a busy road. The staff was frustrated that Harvey would never leave his spot to take part in activities. One day a conversation began that went like this:

>Staff: Why do you sit here all day?
>Harvey replied very quietly: It reminds me of my farm.
>Staff: Tell me about your farm.
>Harvey: I raised flowers and corn for my cows.
>Staff: That sounds like hard work.
>Harvey: Yep!
>Staff: How many cows did you have?
>Harvey: Four hundred and ninety-nine.
>Staff: Four hundred and ninety-nine? Why not an even five hundred?
>Harvey: One got away!

The conversation is amusing, but it makes a serious point. Like the women and their stuffed animals or dolls, like Brian with his list, Harvey liked to do the thing that reminded him of his life when he felt useful.

George and the Usual Suspects

George, a retired sheriff, would come to the activities room, but he would never stay for the activities. As soon as the staff left to gather more residents, George would wander off. One day the activities director brought George into the room where several other residents were already waiting. She said to him, "These are the usual suspects. Could you keep an eye on them while I round up a few more." He replied, "Sure, I can do that."

Men often define themselves by their work. They often feel diminished self-worth when they no longer have their career. This activities director by suggesting an activity that related to George's job, was able to elicit his cooperation, and make him feel useful again. It was a win-win situation for the director and for George.

Suggestions for Interacting

One way to tap into this need to be productive is to ask the facility to provide gardening or woodworking, cooking or sewing opportunities for the residents. Some facilities have charity sales yearly and the residents can sell what they grow, make, knit, or cook and donate the money to a charity of their choice. This gives the residents a real outlet for doing useful work. Staff and family can also reminisce with the residents about what they used to do at work or for their families. People need to be reminded that their lives mattered, that they contributed to the world. It is one of the reasons so many people like to do a life review when they know they are approaching death. They like to talk about the families they raised, the work that they did, the things they accomplished. Writing or taping a family history is a real gift your parent can give to your family. Once she is gone, a piece of family history will also be gone unless it has been preserved.

For a parent with early Alzheimer's, I recommend making a Memory Book. Get pictures of the person, her parents, grandparents, siblings, children, grandchildren, spouse, homes, jobs, and special events. Paste them in a book. Have your parent tell you about the memories each picture elicits. Record the responses and then type them up under each picture. As memory fails, the book makes a great prompt to initiate conversation or jog memory. After the elder is gone, the book provides a wonderful family history for grandchildren or great-grandchildren.

The Power of Music

The Conductor

Mr. Jones was in end-stage Alzheimer's. He didn't speak. He did seem to know his wife, and smiled whenever she came. I was at a loss as to how to reach him when I visited.

Then in a conversation with his wife, she mentioned that he used to like classical music. The next week, I brought a classical tape and a small tape recorder with me. I sat next to his bed and played the music. He arm went up in the air, swaying in time to the music as if he were conducting the orchestra. Once again, I was convinced that music or prayer can reach even those considered unreachable. I began taking music with me and chanting prayers out loud even when visiting comatose people. Does it reach them? I don't know. But it can't hurt!

The Singer

There was a Russian immigrant in a nursing home I visit. He spent most of his days curled up in bed sleeping, or pretending to sleep. No one there speaks Russian or Yiddish, the only two languages he knows. I understand a bit of Yiddish, but I really couldn't speak to him much. But I wanted to reach this sweet, lonely man. Remembering my experience with Mr. Jones, I brought in my tape recorder and a tape of Yiddish folksongs. I turned on the music and he sat up in bed, his eyes shining. His rich, beautiful voice chimed in singing along with the tape. When the song ended, he broke into a torrent of Russian and Yiddish.

Every few sentences I heard a word that I knew, and yet I knew what he was saying. His mother and sister used to sing these songs to him. His mother used to sing in the Yiddish theater. The tape tapped into all the happy memories of his childhood. He sang every song on the tape and I listened appreciatively. Obviously he had been blessed with his mother's singing voice. I had come to bring him pleasure, and found that his singing gave me joy as well.

Suggestions for Interaction

Hearing seems to be the last sense that folks with Alzheimer's or those who are comatose lose. Therefore, music or programs that would interest the resident, and not those that interest the caretaker, should play from time to time in the room. Staff should find out from the family what kind of music or shows the person likes. I am always appalled when I go into a room and the caretaker is blaring loud music that is clearly her taste. Imagine being trapped in a body that can't respond verbally and being constantly assaulted with sounds you hate when you don't have the ability to express your opinion. It is always better to assume the person can hear and choose programs that would soothe.

Bring in music the person used to like and listen to it together. Sing songs to the elder that she used to sing to you, or that were popular in her teenage years.

Holiness and spirituality mean encountering souls where they are. For this reason singing Yiddish songs, listening to classical music, playing gin rummy can be holy soul to soul encounters.

The Power of Choice

Story: I'm Not Your Pet Poodle

Gert was furious when she was taken against her will to the beauty parlor for a haircut. She shouted, "I'm a human being with a mind! I'm not your pet poodle that you take to get bathed and clipped at your convenience. Ask me if I want my hair done!"

Forget that she really looked much better with her hair cut. That was irrelevant to her. What mattered was that she, formerly a strong independent, controlling woman was increasingly not in control of her own life. She could no longer live where she wished, bathe when she wanted, or even get out of bed or go the bathroom when she wanted. All of this was no longer in her control, so she fought vehemently over the "little things" that she could still control: whether to get a haircut, when to take a bath, if she should go to physical therapy, and even if she should have a bedspread on her bed. She desperately needed to feel in control of something in her life. This reaction is particularly strong among people who were fiercely independent and in control of their lives, their family, or their business. The loss of control when they are institutionalized threatens their sense of self. They sometimes try to regain control of the situation by becoming demanding. Unfortunately this often has the adverse effect of antagonizing the staff so that fewer of the resident's demands are met.

Gert railed against the nursing home policy that all residents must get out of bed and sit on a chair for a few hours each day. Granted the nursing home had good reason for this policy. It aided circulation and helped avoid bedsores. But this was less important to her than the aspect of control. She said, "I know when I want to sit and when I want to lie down. I know when I am in pain and when I am tired. Don't presume to tell me what is best for me. I made it to the age of 93 because I know what is best for me."

She added, "Don't tell me I have to get weighed every week. Who cares what I weigh? I'm not running for Miss America!"

Another time I heard this same woman shouting, "Don't tell me to go in my diaper when I have to go to the bathroom. It is bad enough I have to wear this thing, bad enough that I can't get to the bathroom on my own. Don't deny me the dignity of using the toilet because it is inconvenient for you to take me there. And when you don't take me, don't leave me in a wet diaper for half an hour until the next shift arrives."

Residents like this one often antagonize nursing staffs, but I love them. They still have spunk and spirit. They haven't given up on life and they want better from it. Besides, this woman was right. She probably did live to 93 because she knew what was best for her, and it would help for nursing staffs to acknowledge that even when they can't always give in to her demands.

What kinds of compromise can be reached to honor this woman's dignity and still fulfill the requirements of the nursing home? The home requires that all patients get out of bed for a few hours. First explain to your parent the reason for this rule-even if you don't think she will understand. Second, ask if she would prefer to get out of bed in the morning or the afternoon. The same is true of dressing and undressing residents. Some are early risers; others are not. Ask the staff to give your parent the choice of being among the first or last residents dressed. It may be easier for the aides to go down the hall room by room to dress the residents, but that isn't a good enough reason to take control away from the resident. I have heard residents complain about what an aide took out for her to wear. The aide's reply was, "This is what I took out. This is what you will wear." That is unacceptable. Many residents know if they are hot or cold; they know which clothes they like and which they don't. Why can't they choose what they will wear? I know how understaffed most places are. I know how busy the aides are, but how much extra time does it take to ask a resident's opinion? Of course some residents want to wear the same soiled outfit day after day, and the aides cannot allow that, but they could hold up two different clean outfits and ask which one the resident would prefer.

For bathing and hair, some residents never want to wash, and sanitation requires that they must. But again some control can be returned to them by asking whether morning or evening bath time is better or what nightgown the resident wants to wear. Some residents might prefer to wash their hair in the shower rather than going to the beautician. As long as your mother is clean, ask the staff to respect her wishes about how and when she washes.

I know that some aides work hard, but I have also seen groups congregate to talk, ignoring a call button signaling that someone has to go to the bathroom. I have watched a light blink for twenty minutes before I could find someone to aid a resident. That is unacceptable! I have seen residents taken to the bathroom, and left there indefinitely. I know it is an unpleasant job to take a resident to the bathroom or change an adult diaper. I do not envy the aides their job: but it is their job! Family members need to speak up on behalf of all residents, not just their own loved ones, when they see this kind of neglect.

When residents are getting changed, dignity requires that the door be closed or the curtain pulled. Whenever possible, the aide should be the same sex as the resident to avoid embarrassment. By respecting the dignity of the resident, giving choices if possible, and answering bells promptly, staff can make life in a nursing home more tolerable. When you or your parent ask for help, it is inappropriate for a staff member to say, "That's not my job" and walk away. The correct answer is "I will get the person who takes care of that." If the staff is so chronically short-handed that people cannot be dressed, fed, bathed at their convenience, then it is time for you to start looking for another facility. It is your job to be an advocate for your loved one. If this is done in a conversational tone, not a demanding one, you will be more likely to get a positive reaction.

Story: The Two Roses

We choose to see the good or the bad in the world. We choose to see the good or bad in people and situations. We can face the world expecting to find the best, or we can face it expecting to find the worst. And we create the world we live in based on our choice.

I used to visit two women at a particular nursing home. Both were named Rose. Both were mentally sharp but wheelchair bound.

Rose L. chose to sit by the door, outside whenever weather permitted, and greet all the staff, residents and guests who came in and out. We lovingly called her "The Mayor of the Manor." She was the goodwill ambassador for the place. She greeted visitors by name, and asked about their families. She remarked about the helpful staff and the variety of activities in which she constantly remained involved. She was always busy knitting or reading between scheduled activities. She talked about how the staff went out of their way to help her and how glad she was to have prepared meals so she no longer had to cook. She praised her wonderful children who took time to visit her every week.

Rose C. sat outside of her room, waiting to waylay anyone who would listen to her gripe about the inattentive staff, the lack of worthwhile activity and the rotten food. She griped about her ungrateful kids who couldn't be bothered to visit more than once a week.

Both ladies had healthy minds and frail bodies. Both had the same staff, activities and food available. Both had weekly visits from family. Both were telling the truth as they saw it and as they experienced it. But their own choices, their own actions, and their own attitudes were largely responsible for their realities. It is true that the staff was often around Rose L. and avoided Rose C. But what the unhappy lady didn't realize was that by being a faultfinder rather than a joy finder, she created the isolated, hostile, unpleasant environment in which she lived.

The nursing home staff is only human. They will spend more time around those who are pleasant and appreciative and avoid those who are demanding and nasty.

We can choose to be like Rose L. or like Rose C. We are surrounded by good and bad every day. What we choose to focus on, and how we choose to present ourselves to others, will color the kind of world we live in. It is our choice. This is as true for the caregiver as it is for the nursing home resident.

I am not excusing neglect in nursing homes. Every resident deserves to have the bell answered when it is rung, but in places which are chronically short-staffed, when an aide can only take care of one person at a time, the chances are the first one cared for will be the nicer resident. If you can't convince your parent that is in her best interest to be nice to the staff, then do your best to be nice to them for her. Just saying, "I admire you for doing such a difficult, thankless, but necessary job" can work wonders for the staff's morale, particularly when your parent is being difficult. Try to remember to thank them for little extra things they do, and not just to talk to them when there is a problem.

Suggestions for Interaction

Remind your mother that staff will be nicer to her if she is nicer to them. If she has dementia, remind her of this often. When she is not nice to you during a visit, warn her you will leave if her behavior doesn't change-then do it.

If you know your mother is abusive to the staff, occasionally do something thoughtful like baking cookies or send in lunch for the aides. If you can't afford to do that, than make a point of saying something pleasant to the aide whenever you see her. Acknowledge that you know how difficult her job is or how difficult your mother is.

Between Two Worlds

Story: My Husband was Here Last Night

Bella and her husband Vince had been inseparable for nearly 50 years. So great was his love for her that at the age of 90, her husband had quadruple bypass surgery, so he could continue to care for her. But even that love couldn't keep him going forever. I visited Bella days after her beloved husband Vince died. She said, "My husband was here last night." For a moment, I wondered if she had forgotten about his death. But then she continued. "He came back to make sure I am all right. I wanted to go with him, but he said it wasn't my time yet. But he promised he'd be back for me soon." Was she dreaming? Was she hallucinating? Maybe, but I'm not so sure. I do know a few weeks later on the night she died, her niece stayed in the room with her all night. The next day, I spoke to her niece who told me, "I might have been sleeping, but I really thought I was awake last night when for just a second I thought I saw Uncle Vince in the room. I got up and checked on Bella, and she had just died." Was the niece dreaming, or are there loves so strong that they can outlast even death? I prefer to believe Vince really came for Bella as he had promised.

Story: Tell Nina It's a Girl

Sometimes people who are close to death seem to have a foot in both worlds. Nina was eight months pregnant with her first child when her beloved grandmother was dying. Nina hadn't found out the sex of her baby. Nina visited her grandmother often, but on one particular night, Nina was exhausted and had to go home. Nina's mother stayed behind at her mother's bedside. The grandmother whispered, "Tell Nina it's a girl," and then lapsed into final silence. Did her grandmother know or did she guess? Nina's girl, named for her grandmother, was born a few weeks later.

Story: Not Yet

Pauline was dying. All medical indications were that death was imminent. She had lapsed into a coma and no longer responded to the family. The family called me in to pray with them. As I said Viddui, the Jewish Final Confession, for Pauline, her eyes opened wide and she turned to look at me, as if to say "Not yet." One of her children said to me, "I know what she's waiting for. Her anniversary is next week. She's waiting until then to join my father."

How does a dying woman hang on beyond all medically explainable time? How does she even know the date in a comatose state? I don't know, but I do not believe that it was coincidence that Pauline died just moments after her anniversary date arrived.

Suggestions for Interaction

People on the verge of death sometimes seem to have one foot in each world. When you see your dying family member staring at someone/something beyond you, ask who or what she is looking at. And listen to her answer. What she sees may have a reassuring effect on her and on you as she prepares to enter the unknown. Many residents see their beloved spouse or parent in the room waiting to take them to the beyond. If a family member tells you that they see a deceased relative in the room, suspend disbelief. It is pointless to say, "Don't be silly, Mom. You know dad is dead." The vision is comforting to her, and who knows that maybe she sees what you are not yet prepared to see.

If she seems to be hanging on in pain, ask if there is someone or something she is waiting for. Some people are waiting for permission from their family to let go. When someone is suffering, it is a gift to give that permission, even though you don't believe you will ever be able to say the words. One friend managed to say to her ailing husband, "I love you and I will miss you, but I don't want you to suffer. When you are ready, let go. I'll be all right." Shortly thereafter, he passed on.

I've also heard many, many times of families who stayed round the clock at a dying parent's bed side. And then at the one moment when the daughter went to the cafeteria or went to the bathroom, the parent died. Inevitably the family is devastated "that mom died all alone. But it happens so often, I can't help but think that mom couldn't bear to let go when the children were there. She needed that moment alone so she could depart.

The Holiness of Elders

The Eulogy

"I'm sad today. He was a nice man. He was kind to everyone," Ilene, a lovely sweet lady in the middle stages of dementia, said to me as I approached her. Danny was the eighty-nine-year old man of whom she spoke. He had been a long-term resident of an assisted living facility, kind of the elder statesman of the place. He always sat on the front porch, often waiting for his lady friend to pick him up, and greeted all visitors. As the chaplain there, I had come to lead a memorial service for him.

While I waited for the residents to gather, I heard Ilene several times repeating, "I'm sad today. He was a nice man. He was kind to everyone."

During the service, I talked about his intelligence, his kindness, his social activities, and his business acumen. Finally I asked if any residents wanted to speak. Several spoke warmly about him, and then Ilene piped up, "I'm sad today. He was a nice man. He was kind to everyone."

The service continued, punctuated periodically by "I'm sad today. He was a nice man. He was kind to everyone." Others looked at her, annoyed, and tried to hush her up, but I was touched by her eulogy, repeated almost like a mantra.

And I really believe when Danny goes before the Throne of Judgment, the words God will weigh most heavily in his favor are the words from a broken life he touched, "I'm sad today. He was a nice man. He was kind to everyone."

This story is proof that kindness matters, especially to those with Alzheimer's. In fact, feelings remain when almost everything else is lost. People, even in end stage Alzheimer's, even when they no longer can speak, will still react to a gentle touch, a smile, a kind word, and they will still get agitated by noise, harsh treatment, or unkind words.

Suggestions for Interaction

When you visit a parent with dementia, bring your patience with you. I know how frustrating it is to answer the same question twenty times or listen to the same story over and over. But she is trying to communicate with you, and for her each time she tells the story or asks the question, it is the first time.

You can try to change the subject, or show her a photo album, or put on music, or polish her nails, or put lotion on her hands, or ask her if she wants to go for a walk. Sometime these distractions will get her out of the repetitive loop.

Sabbath Candles

"The dimly burning wick shall he not quench." (Isaiah 42:3)

It was Friday afternoon, and the Jewish nursing home residents filled the activity room for Sabbath services. I lit the Sabbath candles-two tapers of the same size, lit from the same match. Yet one candle burned with a large orange flame and the other produced a minute, barely visible flicker of blue. "That one isn't lit," called out several of the residents. I looked again and saw that the blue flicker was still barely visible. I said the blessings, and as always I felt the spirit of the Sabbath fill the room as the residents joined me in singing *Shalom Aleichem, Peace to You.*

But my eyes kept going back to those two candles, the one blazing; the other just flickering. When it came time for my sermon, I threw out what I had prepared, and talked instead about those candles. It occurred to me that those candles were a metaphor for humanity. All of us were given the same spark of divinity from the same Source. Yet some let that spark shine forth and brighten the world; others squelch the soul-light until it is almost extinguished. They show nothing of their soul-light to the world.

After flickering through most of the service, the little light suddenly burst into full flame. And that too was a metaphor for humanity. No matter how dark out lives have been, no matter how hard we have tried to extinguish our soul-light, it never goes out completely. And with repentance and change of heart, it is never too late, to let God's light within us shine and brighten the world.

I think the metaphor of the candles is particularly appropriate for the nursing home residents. For some of them, in pain, frail, forgetful, life must seem like that flickering blue candle, but for a moment, during Sabbath services, when they join in prayer, the life and the soul blaze forth brightly again.

I think again of Dr. Fishman, the silent man in the end stage of Alzheimer's, who broke his silence to say "Good Shabbas." I realized that for that one brief moment, I had seen a flicker again become a flame. And that is why life, even when it is reduced to a flicker, is so precious. That is why I love my work as a geriatric chaplain. I am sometimes given the blessing of seeing the divine spark shine forth from "the dimly burning wick."

Suggestions for Interaction

Look for the moments of holiness in even the simplest interaction with a family member who has Alzheimer's. React to the emotions you see conveyed in the face or body language. Say, "You look happy/sad/ today. Can you tell me why?" If she can't speak, tell her family news that will make her happy. Assume she can hear and understand you even if she can't respond.

If your relationship with your parent has not been a good one, sometimes the time spent together at the end of life can be a healing one-if you can get past any resentment or anger you feel at the person she was, and try to just see and interact with the person she is now. Even if you cannot heal the relationship, when she dies, she can comfort yourself knowing you did the best you could. You also teach a powerful lesson to your children that the commandment to "honor your father and mother" does not come with the caveat "If you think they deserve it."

Do Not Go Gentle?

In the poem *Do Not Go Gentle into that Good Night*, Dylan Thomas tells his father "to rage against the dying of the light."

This is a son's poem to his father, but this sentiment often represents the attitude of the young, not the old.

Some elderly who have lost too many loved ones, have debilitating diseases like ALS or Parkinson's, or suffer from chronic pain, really do just want to "go gentle into that good night." In such cases, the hardest and greatest gift a child can give the parent is to obey the parent's end of life directives.

If there is a living will, and most nursing homes require one, you should honor it. Often a parent will hang on in agony to a life she no longer wants because of the prayers and pleas of the children. In such cases, these pleas are impediments to the dying process. In the Talmud, there is the story of Judah the Prince whose students were praying outside of his window. The prayers prevented him from dying. A servant woman, seeing Judah's agony, shattered a pot. The noise startled the students who momentarily stopped praying. In that instant, Judah died. The Talmud considered the servant a worthy woman. While the law forbids hastening death, it doesn't require that we create artificial barriers to postpone the inevitable. In the story, the students meant well. But they were only postponing the inevitable and keeping their master alive in great pain. The servant woman loved the master enough to remove the barrier that was prolonging his death.

The selfless thing for you to do when a parent is dying in great pain is to give the parent permission to let go. You can say something like, "I love you. I will miss you, but I will be okay. I know that you will always be with me in spirit. So if you are in too much pain or too weak to fight any longer, it is all right if you let go (or go to God)." I know several people who told me they could never say they words. But then when they saw their loved one struggling in agony for each breath, they found the courage and the love to give their loved one permission to let go.

Of course, you cannot help them go. That is crossing over into God's realm. There is often a fine line between what is permissible for a dying patient and what is not. The key is often intent. For example, you may request additional morphine to relieve the pain of your loved one, even if that dosage might hasten the dying, but intentionally giving the person a large dosage to cause death is not allowed. Families and doctors struggle with this balance every day.

But while you aren't permitted to end life, you also need not prolong death. Families and physicians should do everything possible to give every minute to those who wish to "rage against the dying of the light." But they can avoid breathing tubes, dialysis, resuscitation orders, and even feeding tubes to honor the wishes of those who are ready to "go gentle into that good night."

I Want to Die

When visiting the sick or elderly, I often hear, "I'm suffering. I want to die." And truthfully, in the face of so much suffering, I've often struggled to find a response. So I was quite surprised in *Numbers* 11:14-16 to find Moses say to God, "This burden is too heavy for me. If you will deal with me so, kill me, I pray."

Interestingly, God doesn't berate Moses for those feelings or question his right to make such a request. God doesn't shout at Moses, "Life is a gift I gave you. How dare you reject my gift?" And God doesn't remove the burdens that Moses faces.

God does tell Moses to gather others in the community "that they shall bear the burden with you; that you bear it not yourself alone." (*Numbers* 11:17) God's answer to Moses and to us is: when you are suffering, ask for help. Get yourself a support system so that you don't bear your burdens alone. This is good advice not only for your ailing parent but also for you who are bearing the burden of caring for her.

That's why we are commanded to visit the sick and the elderly. In doing so, we share their burdens with them and help reduce the suffering.

The lesson from this is that it is okay to rail against suffering and to question the value of life; it is even okay to question God. As God listened to Moses, God will listen to all who call out in pain. However, God didn't give Moses what he asked for, but what he needed. We have to understand when we or our loved ones are suffering, God may not give us relief from pain or an early death, but God will give us what we need, the strength, the courage, the support to bear our burdens. When we stand together with those who suffer, we stand on holy ground and we do holy work. You, as a child of a dying parent, have a real opportunity, albeit a difficult one to respect you parent's last wishes, even when they contradict what you want.

When we hear a parent say, "I want to die," it is crucial that you hear and acknowledge the pain and the losses behind the words. Saying, "Don't say that. You have a lot to live for" will shut down communication. Finding out why she wants to die may open up communication. Does she wish to escape pain? Is she depressed? Does she feel like a burden? Does she wish to join loved ones who have died? Is she afraid of financially ruining your family with an extended life? Is she afraid of having nothing left to leave you if she lives too long? Does she feel lonely and abandoned? Does she hate feeling dependent? For some of these reasons, there may be solutions. Pain can be managed by a staff and physicians who are willing to make the effort. You can be her advocate to the medical staff if she is in obvious pain.

Many elders are under the mistaken impression that the parent's money is the children's inheritance. Some parents would rather die or do without needed care than spend their children's inheritance. If you can help her to think of her money as *her money*, then she may be willing to spend it to care for herself. Again this requires you to put your best interests on hold to do what is in her best interest. Isn't that the essence of *honor your father and mother?*

Religious groups, volunteers, chaplains and staff can ease the loneliness if your family cannot or will not do so.

For some issues, like wishing to join loved ones, a solution is more difficult. Sometimes encouraging your mother to show pictures or talk about the loved one helps; other times that just brings back painful memories. In any case, it is not necessary to solve the problems that lead her to wish for death; but it is crucial to *hear* them. It is not necessary to be a good problem solver; it is essential to be a good listener. Sometimes after your mother knows that her feelings have been heard and validated, it is possible to get her to think about what she still has to live for, to be thankful for. But it is also important to realize that sometimes she really is worn out and ready to die. While you may not help her fulfill this wish to die, you can sometimes help just by listening to it.

Broken Vessels

"Cast me not off in the time of old age; when my strength
faileth, forsake me not."
—(Psalm 7:19)

The Bible says that God lovingly carved the letters of the Ten Commandments into the two tablets of stone. Then Moses came down from the mountain, saw the Israelites with the golden calf, and threw the tablets down in anger, smashing them. Later a second set of tablets was inscribed by God. When Moses brought down these second tablets, and placed them in the arc, legend says, he scooped up the pieces of the broken tablets and placed them in the arc as well. The reason given is that a thing that is holy remains holy, even when it is broken.

I contend that the same is true of people. People are holy because they contain the soul, the holy spark, and because they are created in the divine image. They remain holy even when they are broken, either physically or mentally, whether by genetics, birth, accident, injury or age-related conditions. Someone who is not physically or mentally perfect is still holy. We honor God's holiness and our own when we continue to honor the holiness in all people regardless of their physical or mental state.

It therefore, offends the holiness of comatose people to be described as "vegetables" in a "persistent vegetative state." It honors their holiness if we touch their hand or talk to them lovingly. Whether or not we believe that they can hear us, God can hear us and I believe that God is a loving parent who rejoices in seeing others treating God's children with love.

I often hear people say that they cannot visit hospitals or nursing homes. It frightens them, it depresses them, and it reminds them of what they may become someday. As someone who spends her days in nursing homes and hospitals, I really do understand those fears. But I also understand that the people in those places are also afraid and depressed, and those visits are what make their days bearable. And while I do fear ending up in one of those places myself, if I do, I hope people I love will still visit me.

Story: The Old man and the Wheelbarrow

An old man lived with his son, daughter-in-law and grandchildren. The family complained that the old man used up vital resources without contributing anything to the family. Finally the son decided that his father must die so the rest of the family could prosper. The son built a wheelbarrow, put his father in it, and wheeled it to the top of a mountain. As he got ready to push the wheelbarrow, with his father in it, over the cliff, his father said to him, "Throw me over, but save the wheelbarrow. Your children will need it someday for you."

The truth is our children learn by what we do. If we show love, respect and compassion to our parents, that is what our children will learn. But if we show fear, anger, and resentment, that is what our children will learn.

Some people say I would visit, but I don't know what to do. S/he can't communicate. However, I have found when there are no words or the words make no sense, it is possible to relate to the feelings conveyed by facial expressions and body language and make contact "soul to soul." It is possible to put fear and discomfort aside when you come to these encounters looking for the holy in the other person.

Top Questions/Comments by Nursing Home Residents

1.   I want to go home. Why can't I go home?

First recognize that the reference to home is ambiguous. What **home** are they thinking about?-the residence where they most recently lived? The home where they lived with their spouse and maybe raised their family? Their childhood home? Or the Eternal Home to which we will all go eventually?

There is little to gain in telling them they can't go home, or their home was sold, or the facility they are in is home now. Don't try to explain that they can no longer live alone; they rarely recognize the severity of their impairments and they no longer accept abstract concepts anyway.

You might try to ask them to talk about their home, what they loved best about their home. Then at least you will know which home they are missing. If it helps rather than agitates, you can talk about your memories of that home, too. Another alternative is to say: I'm sorry you don't like it here. I'll try to find another place for you but it will take some time to make other arrangements. Or you can say: you are here to get treatment for your memory, hearing, vision, broken hip, etc. When you get well, we can talk about going home. You might even specify what the person would have to be able to do: We can talk about your going home when you can walk by yourself, do your cooking and laundry, etc. (even though you expect this will never happen). This last approach won't work with people in early stages of dementia because they still believe they can care for themselves.

2.   I want my mother. She must be wondering where I am.

Little will be gained by saying the mother is dead. It will make the person experience grief as if the death had just occurred and it will also make her feel guilty for not remembering. Better to say: let's look for her together; then take her for a walk. If you feel that is deceitful and you are uncomfortable with that approach, say: Can you tell me your favorite memories of your mother? Or you as the child or grandchild can say: My favorite memory of Grandmom is . . . Or ask: Do you remember how much she loved to cook? Are you hungry now? Let's find you something to eat or ask: What was your favorite recipe of hers? Do you remember how she liked to garden. Why don't we take a walk in the garden? Sometimes these distractions will work. Ask her the best advice her mother ever gave her and then ask what advice she would give you or her grandchildren. In short the strategy is to evoke a pleasant memory and then offer a diversion. Keep in mind that a person with progressing dementia has a short memory span and a diversion may turn her attention to other topics.

3.   Where is my husband or wife?

Saying the person is too ill to visit or is dead will create a negative emotional reaction. However, if a spouse visited daily, then passed away, the person should be told at least once; otherwise she will miss her spouse, experience grief, anxiety, or distress, and not be able to verbalize why she has those feelings. If you are comfortable entering the time zone the resident is in (which is the time when the spouse was alive), you can say: he's probably in the den reading or in the garage tinkering with the car(whatever the spouse would have been doing in his free time.) If entering their time zone feels dishonest to you, then you could ask them to talk to you about the spouse. E.g: How did you meet dad? What was dad like when he was younger? What did(do) you like best about dad?

4.   Where is my family? I need to get back to them.

Remind her that you are there and reassure her that everyone in the family knows where she is. Tell her about family members living out of town or away at school. Tell her others are working/ caring for children/ in school. Say they love her and miss her and will visit as soon as they can. Save cards from out-of-town relatives to read to her again when she asks for them.

The person may show surprise that "Bill" who she still thinks of as a child, is in college or married. You can have a discussion about "how time flies" or "how fast children grow up." Bring up old family stories, sayings, memories relating to the person she is asking for. Invoking true family stories bring positive feelings and offer a diversion.

5. I want to die. Why can't the Lord take me?

Do not argue. Do not tell her she doesn't mean it because she does. If she is religious, you can say "God will call you when it is your time," or it's not for us to choose when it is our time," or "Your job on earth must not be done yet."

6. I feel useless. I'm too old/sick to do anything anymore.

Suggest things they can still do: record/tell family stories for younger generation, call someone who is ill, talk with others in the facility who are lonely, pray for others/peace/country. Also remind her that we are human beings not human doings and that you and God love her just the way she is.

7. I don't belong here with all these sick, old people.

Residents rarely recognize the degree of physical or mental impairment they have, particularly in the early stages of decline. They don't empathize, but rather seem revolted by others physically or mentally worse off than themselves. But this is a reaction born of fear. At some level they are afraid that that is what they too will become.

8. Why can't you do my laundry, shopping, hair etc.?

People who were never selfish before, as they get frailer, may become selfish. People who were already self-centered will only become more so as they become sick or frail. As their world is increasingly out of their control, they need to feel in control of something, and frequently they take this out on those they love or who love them the most. Joan was in the middle of chemotherapy when her mother asked if Joan could start doing the mother's laundry! It hurts when the parent who was always your protector suddenly puts herself first, above your health needs. But again remember that she is acting out of fear. Do not take on additional tasks that will be a burden to you. Tell her: I am not well enough/home enough to do that now, but if a time comes when I can do it, I will. When she sends you on an errand, do not promise to do it immediately. Say: "I'll do my best to get that for you" or, "I am very busy at work today, but I will get it as soon as I can." If she gets overly demanding or abusive, tell her you will see her next week, but you must leave now-then do it.

9.   Someone stole my ring/teeth/ hearing aid.

The sad truth is that sometimes things do disappear in nursing homes, but often as not the resident has misplaced the item. It is less painful for the person to say (and believe) that the item was stolen than to admit that she doesn't remember where she put it. Say: "Let me help you look for that" and then search the room together. Ask laundry staff to check-sometimes an item was left in a pocket and turns up in the laundry. Ask dietary to look on the meal trays. Carol's aunt used to leave her dentures in her coffee cup! If you do not find the item, do report it to the staff as lost or missing-not as stolen. Most facilities have a lost and found, usually at the reception desk or nursing station. Sometimes residents wonder into the wrong room and pick things up. If you see another resident with the missing item, report it to staff and let them get it for you. Do not leave money or items of real or sentimental value in the room. Most facilities have a safe for valuables, although I strongly recommend that family keep real valuables with them. Many facilities also have an account set up where residents can leave money at the office or receptionist's desk, and come to get it when they need it.

10. Who's paying for the meals/hair, other services? I can't afford this.

Our parents' generation, the Depression survivors have a real fear of running out of money which may or may not have any basis in the reality of their financial situation. Many from this generation are ashamed or reluctant to accept anything they perceive as charity. Make it clear that they are paying for their care. Tell them: "Your insurance covers it" or "Social Security pays for it," or "It's all taken care of from your savings"; or "it's included in your rent; don't worry about it." If assets such as stock, an insurance policy, or a home were sold to pay, decide whether or not to tell them depending on how mentally aware they are, how attached to these items they were, and whether or not the possible sale of these items had been discussed in the past. For most of their generation, the home was their security, and knowing it was sold will increase their anxiety. For many the insurance policy was the legacy they invested in for their children. Telling them it had to be cashed in to pay their expenses will just upset them. The best way to guarantee that your parent won't run out of money is to choose an assisted living/nursing home that agrees to accept Social Security and Medicare/Medicaid as payment when all other money runs out. These places usually require that the parent/ children guarantee fees for 2-3 years. If the parent outlives that time and their money, the facility will then accept the Social Security check as payment.

11. Where are my social Security or pension checks? I'm not getting them. Someone is/you are stealing my money.

The easiest thing to say is that the checks are automatically deposited or they are used to pay for their rent and meals.

12. They hit me/hurt me/ are mean to me.

This is every caregiver's nightmare. Often the resident has misinterpreted the actions of staff. A good facility will call whenever there is any kind of incident that leads to injury. If you have not been called, and she has bruises, ask the staff what happened.

People with dementia often imagine violence. I heard one woman say that her roommate had taken her cross off the wall and beat her with it-but the cross was still on the wall, and there were no signs of injury. However, do not ignore such complaints because residents do sometimes hurt each other, and staff sometimes can be mean. Is she complaining about all staff or residents, or one particular person?

Report her complaints to staff (not the person she is complaining about), and ask if there have been any other complaints about this resident or staff member.

Some residents become abusive to staff. Some resist necessary hygiene activities such as baths and must be coerced. If a staff member grabs a resident's arm gently to keep from getting hit, this could leave faint bruising on the thin skin of an elderly person, especially if she is taking blood thinners such as coumadin. But again, an event such as this should be reported to you as soon as it happens. Whenever there is a question of abuse, report it to the charge nurse. If you are not satisfied with the result, talk to the Director of

Nursing or the administrator. If after your investigation, or after talking to other families, you still feel uneasy, contact the state or county Ombudsman and report the situation. This person is trained to help families deal with care-giving issues. Whether they are state employees or volunteers, their training is extensive. The phone number or e-mail for the ombudsman should be posted around the facility at the nurses' station, common rooms, or activity rooms. Most facilities have a professional working relationship with the Ombudsman and will cooperate with him/her.

13. I don't want to take a bath/ change my clothes/ get my hair washed.

The older generation is more modest. The problem could be as simple as a female not wanting a male aide to bathe her or a male resident not wanting to bathe in front of a female aide. Ask staff to honor modesty of residents as much as possible. It might be that staff has decided to bathe someone at 8:00 at night when the resident is a morning person who is exhausted by evening. Staff often wants things done at their convenience, not the convenience of the resident. Facilities would do well to remind staff that the residents pay their salaries and they deserve some accommodation. Ask staff to give back some control to your parent. For dressing, suggest that they show your mother two outfits and ask which one she would like to wear. If she balks at bathing in the morning, ask staff to ask her if she would prefer to bathe in the afternoon or the evening. I know staff doesn't like this, but a good facility will put the preferences of the resident over the convenience of the aide. If she balks at going to the hairdresser, perhaps you can schedule an appointment for her when you can go with her, and make it a mother-daughter outing. Another alternative is to make washing her hair part of her bath. Most residents who are approached with kindness, humor, and respect rather than with impatience and demands can be coaxed to do what they need to do.

14. I don't want that _____(insert racial, religious, or sexist epithet) in my room.

Dealing with racist, insulting, nasty, aggressive words or behavior aimed at staff or at you is exceedingly difficult. Biases that were kept inside when the impulse control portion of the brain worked properly will spill out now. You may be appalled at what your parent says or does, but trying to be logical with her and explaining how offensive her words/ actions are rarely works. You wouldn't expect someone with a broken leg to walk; you can't expect someone with a broken brain to think or act logically. You can go out of your way to apologize/ treat the staff member with the respect due, but you can't do anything about your parent's behavior.

You can tell her that what she said or did was offensive to the staff member and to you, and that she needs the help of the staff, but this rarely has more than a short-term effect.

When she is nasty, or guilt-provoking with you, do not allow her to push your buttons. Tell her you love her, but you will not stay to take her abuse. Tell her you hope she is in a better frame of mind when you return on (name day). Then leave!

15. Mother cries when you come.

Ask her: "I can see you are upset. Can you tell me why you are crying?"

Do not say: "Mom, stop crying. This is ridiculous." It is important to acknowledge her feelings even if you don't understand them. Is it the anniversary of the death of someone she loved? I can't explain how residents with dementia know when it is a special day, but sometimes, somehow, they do.

Talk to staff. Did something happen to upset her? Has she been agitated all day? Was there a change in her routine that day? Is it a full moon? (Don't laugh!) Staff will attest to the fact that some residents become agitated during a full moon. Ask staff how she acted before you came. Did she attend activities? Sometimes crying when you are there is just a subtle form of emotional blackmail to evoke guilt, and she may be happy and active when you leave.

16. I fell today and nobody helped me.

Check with staff to see if she did fall. Check for bruises. Ask her where she hurts. If she did fall, and you were not notified, find out why. You should be called anytime there is any kind of incident involving your parent. There will always be a risk of falls with this population. If your parent is at high risk for falls, find out what precautions the place can take. Physical restraint is illegal in most states. However, the facility can put an alarm on the wheelchair to alert them when she tries to stand. It can provide a cane or walker. The facility can put sides/guardrails on the bed, or lower the bed, and it should always have grab bars in bathrooms. Staff should be told to watch out for residents who often forget to use their canes or walkers.

17. There's nothing to do here or No one ever tells me what is going on here.

Every facility has as activity department and a monthly calendar of events. Most facilities will provide a copy of it to interested families. Very often programs are also announced over the P.A. system. But Alzheimer's residents may not remember. In good facilities, staff should come around right before an activity to bring residents to the event. Family is usually invited to attend as well. Good facilities also keep a record of who attends what activity. If you are concerned, ask to see which events your parent has attended. Also tell staff if there are activities that would be of special interest to your parent so they can be sure to gather her/him for those events. Most places have activities planned for most holidays because residents often can't travel to be with their family.

Remember that it is easier to complain than to admit that she can't read/has lost the calendar of events. Also remember that often residents don't remember that they have attended an activity. Finally remember the Resident Bill of Rights gives residents the right to refuse to attend activities.

18. My memory is so bad.

There is nothing sadder than hearing that from someone in early Alzheimer's who is aware enough to know that they are forgetting people, places, words, and things they should remember. Acknowledge the confusion, fear and sense of loss that comes with a failing memory. "That's scary/ frustrating, isn't it?" Empathize if you also sometimes have 'senior moments.' "I hate when that happens to me. The older I get, the more I seem to forget." Calm them. "Don't try so hard to remember. Sometimes I find a lost memory or word comes back to me when I stop trying to remember it." If possible, direct them to a different subject.

SUPPLEMENTAL READINGS

by Carol Kasser

With apologies to Dylan Thomas, my poem for those dying and ready to go is

Go Gently into that Good Night

Go gently, beloved into that good night
Old age may go in peace at close of day
Rest, rest, in God's Eternal Light.

I'm Not Afraid

I'm not afraid my life will end
for death comes gently, as a friend.
I'll slip softly into life's ebb and flow,
for into God's loving hands I'll go.
Do not fear that I'll be alone.
God is with me; I am God's own.
As I leave, all pain will cease.
I'll go at last to God's world of peace.
I will not fret for you my love.
You'll find comfort from above.
Nor will I fear while we're apart.
I'll live on in your loving heart.
When your earthly bonds set you free,
You'll come to rejoin your God . . . and me.

Let my Life Be My Prayer

When my voice cannot, let my life sing to You,
a song of faith, of joy, of love,
of gratitude, compassion, caring, hope.
When my words or my voice fail me,
let my life stand before you as my prayer.

Knit Your Love

It is possible to knit your love
And stitch together a life
And that is what you did for us
As a loving parent, grandmom, wife.
You could use your golden hands
To fashion art from thread,
Or to cuddle all the young ones,
And bake for them cakes or bread.
And when you sewed a garment
more than a coat, a scarf, a glove,
you put your hopes and dreams inside
and stitched for us your love.

I Think of Her

I think of her on a summer day
when the sun shines bright and children play.
I think of her when leaves turn gold,
when days are crisp, and evenings cold.
I think of her during winter white
when the day is chilled, and too long the night.
I think of her when flowers bloom
and the warm air fills with sweet perfume.
I think of her when I am sad,
when I am lonely, and life seems bad.
I think of her with joy to share
and I want to call, but she's not there.

I think of her often now that we're apart;
but her spirit lives on in my loving heart.

A Breathing Meditation for Healing

(breathe in and out deeply and slowly)
Breathe in healing, breathe out fear.
Breathe in peace, breathe out pain.
Breathe in love, breathe our anger.
Breathe in forgiveness, breathe out grudges.
Breathe in comfort, breathe out sorrow.
Breath in serenity, breathe out stress.
Breathe in healing, breathe out fear.
Breathe in peace, breathe out pain.

For those Living and Dying With Alzheimer's

The disease takes away my memories.
It takes away my control.
But let it never touch my spirit.
Let it never touch my soul.
It may ravage all my body
and play tricks upon my mind;
but despite it all and through it all,
may I stay gentle, sweet and kind.

Those Eyes

I look into those empty eyes.
Today you aren't there.
I do not see your soul now,
just a wide-eyed vacant stare.
I used to feel so safe
beneath their watchful glance.
Those eyes used to sparkle;
those eyes used to dance.

Those eyes used to light with joy
when I would score a goal.
Now those eyes don't know me;
It's like looking in a hole.
Those are eyes that loved me,
that used to glow with pride;
Now I feel like an orphan
though I'm standing by your side.
Sometimes there's a glimmer,
a momentary spark.
For that moment, my mom is home,
but then those eyes go dark.
Those eyes have no memories
of the love they used to give.
So my memories must speak for you
as long as we both shall live.

After a death From Alzheimer's

We are not here to mourn a death, but to celebrate a life.

Over the past few years, we saw our friend die by inches. Those who loved her have already mourned each little loss, each little death, each lost ability, each lost memory. Now she is free of that terrible illness that took her away from herself and those who loved her, one piece at a time.

In the past few years, Alzheimer's took away many of her memories; fortunately it could not take away our memories of her.

It took away her strength and independence, but not the lesson of strength and independence she had taught by her example.

It took away her desire to do the things she once loved to do, but not our memories of the loving things she did for us.

It took away her ability to care for other, but not the legacy of caring we learned by knowing her.

Alzheimer's victory was shallow and temporary. Once more she is in a place where she can watch over those she loves. And those she loves are in a place where they can remember her as she once was: vibrant, strong, caring and loving.

Here's to the Lonely

Here's to the lonely, the forgotten, the ill
God loved them always, God loves them still.
For those who feel friendless, for those who may cry,
"No one will care if I live or I die."
This I am sure of, this they should know,
heaven awaits those ignored down below.

So What?
By Joan Phillips

There is a nice lady sorting my laundry in my room.
Is it my daughter or my mother?
So what? I feel her love.
I think I went to a class today.
Was it exercise or crafts?
So what? I helped and I felt proud.
Yesterday I'm told I went to church.
Was it Catholic, Protestant, or Jewish?
So what? I felt the love.
This afternoon a lady with a dog came to visit.
Who they are I don't know.
So what? I love dogs.
A nice girl came in to read to me.
She's always around and greets everyone with a smile.
Does she work here? Is she a volunteer?
So what? I feel her love.
A cute young man came to see me.
He stops a lot to visit.
He told me a funny story.
Who he is or why he visits, I don't know.
So what? I feel his concern.
There are people here to see me.
They are singing my favorite songs and hymns.
Are they my family? Are they from my church?

So what? I feel their love.
There's a bright light or a glow.
A dove tells me I must go.
So what? I am ready to feel GOD'S LOVE.

Holy Readings for Aging Wisely

Bless the Lord, O my soul;
And all that is within me bless God's holy name.
Bless the Lord, O my soul,
And forget not all of God's benefits;
Who forgives all your iniquity;
Who heals all your diseases;
Who redeems your life from the pit;
Who encompasses you with loving-kindness and tender mercies;
Who satisfies your old age with good things
So that your youth is renewed like an eagle. (*Psalm 103:1-5*)

We bring our years to an end as a tale that is told.
The days of our lives are three score and ten,
or even by reason of strength four score years;
Yet is their pride but travail and vanity;
for it is speedily gone, and we fly away.
Who knows the power of Your anger,
and Your wrath according to the awe that is due unto You?
So teach us to number our days,
that we may get us a heart of wisdom. (*Psalm 90:9-12*)

The righteous shall flourish like a palm tree;
and grow mighty like the cedar in Lebanon.
Planted in the house of the Lord,
they shall bring forth fruit in old age;
they shall be full of sap and richness;
to declare that the Lord is upright,
my Rock, in whom there is no unrighteousness. (*Psalm 92:13-16*)

Cast thy burdens upon the Lord, and God will sustain you.
God will never suffer the righteous to be moved. (*Psalm 55:23*)

Hallelujah!
Praise God in the sanctuary.
Give praise in the firmament of God's power.
Give praise according to God's abundant greatness.
Give praise with the blast of the horn.
Give praise with the psaltery and the harp.
Give praise with the timbrel and the dance.
Give praise with stringed instruments and the pipe.
Praise God with cymbals banging.
Give praise with cymbals clanging.
Let every soul praise God. Hallelujah. (*Psalm 150*)

Set a guard, O God to my mouth;
keep watch at the door of my lips.
Incline not my heart to do any evil thing. (*Psalm 141:3-4*)

These are the obligations without measure
whose reward too is without measure:
To honor father and mother;
To perform kind and loving deeds;
To attend the house of prayer daily;
To welcome the stranger;
To visit the sick;
To rejoice with bride and groom;
To honor the dead and console the bereaved;
To pray with sincerity;
To make peace where there is discord;
And the study of God's laws is equal to them all
because it leads to them all. (Adapted from daily Jewish prayer)

Happy are they that keep justice,
that do righteousness at all times. (*Psalm 106:3*)

Hear O Israel, the Lord our God, the Lord is one.
You shall love the Lord you God with all your heart,
with all your soul and with all your might.
And these words that I command you this day
shall be upon your heart. You shall teach them

diligently unto your children, and you shall speak of them
when you sit in your home, when you walk by the way,
when you lie down and when you rise up.
they shall be for frontlets between your eyes.
You shall write then upon the doorposts of your home
and upon your gates. (*Deuteronomy 6:4-9*)

You are the light of the world . . . Let your light so shine before men
That they may see your good works and give glory to your Father who is in
heaven. (*Matthew 5:14. 16*)

You shall love your neighbor as yourself. (*Leviticus: 19:18* and *Mark 12:31*)

In the Morning

This is the day the Lord has made.
Rejoice and be glad in it. (*Psalm 118:24*)

I am grateful to You Living and Eternal Ruler,
For You have returned my soul within me with compassion,
Abundant is your faithfulness. (Jewish morning prayer)

Our father who art in heaven
Hallowed be thy name
Thy kingdom come, thy will be done
On earth as it is in heaven
Give us this day our daily bread;
And forgive us our trespasses
As we forgive those who trespass against us.
And lead us not into temptation,
But deliver us from evil. (*Matthew 6:9-13*)

The world is new to us every morning.
This is God's gift;
And every human being
should feel reborn every day. (Baal Shem Tov)

In the Evening

Blessed are You, O God, Ruler of the universe
Who makes the bands of sleep to fall upon my eyes,
And slumber upon my eyelids.
May it be your will, O God, that I lie down in peace,
and let me rise up again in peace.
Let my thoughts not trouble me,
nor evil dreams, nor evil desires.
But let my rest be perfect before You. (Jewish evening prayer)

Now I lay me down to sleep,
I pray the Lord my soul to keep
If I should die before I wake,
I pray the Lord my soul to take.
(Children's evening prayer)

I lay me down and I sleep;
I awake for the Lord sustains me.
I am not afraid. (*Psalm 3:6-7*)

In peace will I both lay me down and sleep;
For You, Lord, make me dwell alone in safety. (*Psalm 4:9*)

For you do light my lamp;
The Lord my God does lighten my darkness. (*Psalm 18:29*)

In Illness

Be gracious unto me, O Lord,
For I languish away.
Heal me, O Lord, for my bones are frightened,
My soul is sorely afraid;
And thou, O Lord, how long?
Return O Lord, deliver my soul
Save me for Your mercy's sake. (*Psalm 6:3-5*)

As for me I will call upon God;
And the Lord will heal me. (*Psalm 55:17*)

Heal me, O Lord, and I shall be healed.
Save me and I shall be saved.
For You are my praise. (*Jeremiah 17:14*)

May it be your will O Lord
Speedily to send me perfect healing from heaven,
Healing of body and healing of soul
along with all those who are sick. (Adaptation of Jewish healing prayer).

For Specific Ailments

Blessed is the Eternal God who has implanted mind and instinct in every human being.
Blessed is the Eternal God who opens the eyes of the blind.
Blessed is the Eternal God whose power lifts up the fallen.
Blessed is the Eternal God who makes firm each person's steps.
Blessed is the eternal God who gives strength to the weary.
(adapted from Jewish morning blessings)

The Lord will give strength unto His people.
The Lord will bless His people with peace. (*Psalm 29:11*)

Cast me not off in the time of my old age.
When my strength fails, forsake me not. (*Psalm 71:9*)

When you are old, I am still the same,
When your hair is gray, I will support you.
I have made, and I will bear,
Yes, I will carry and I will save you.
(adapted from *Isaiah 46:4*)

For with You is the fountain of life;
In Your light do we see light. (*Psalm 36:10*)

Blessed is the Eternal God Creator of the Universe
Who has made our bodies with wisdom
Combining veins, arteries and organs into a finely balanced network (or literally-creating many openings and cavities)
So that if any one of them failed life could not be sustained.
Wondrous Fashioner and Sustainer of life, Source of our health and our strength, we give You thanks and praise. (Jewish Morning Prayer)

Be gracious unto me, O Lord
for I am in distress.
Mine eye wastes away with vexation,
Yea, my body and my soul.
For my life is spent in sorrow, and my years in sighing;
My strength fails . . . and my bones are wasted away.
Because of all my adversities, I have become a reproach,
Yea, unto my neighbors exceedingly, and to my acquaintances.
They that see me without flee from me;
I am forgotten as a dead man out of mind.
I am like a useless vessel . . .
But as for me, I have trusted in You, O Lord,
I have said "You are my God."
My times are in Your hand;
Deliver me . . . (*Psalm 31:10-16*)

Why are you cast down O my soul?
And why do you moan within me?
Hope in God, for I shall yet praise Him,
the salvation of my countenance and my God. (*Psalm 43:5*)

The spirit of man will sustain his infirmity,
but a broken spirit who can bear? (*Proverbs 18:14*)

When Dissatisfied With Your Body

For you have made my reins;
You did knit me together in my mother's womb.

I will give thanks unto You
for I am fearfully and wonderfully made.
Wonderful are Your works;
and this my soul knows right well. (*Psalm 139:13-14*)

Healing Prayer for Others

Heal her now O God I beseech You. (*Numbers 12:13*)

God, preserve him and keep him alive,
Let him be called happy in the land;
And deliver him not unto his enemies.
God support him in his bed of illness,
May you turn away all his lying down in sickness.
As for me I have said, "O God, be gracious unto me,
Heal my soul." (*Psalm 41:3-5*)

After Healing or Surviving a Dangerous Situation

O Lord my God, I cried unto You, and You did heal me.
Lord, You saved me from the risk of death, You kept me alive."
(*Psalm 30:3-4*)

Your vows are upon me God;
I will render thanksgiving to You.
For you have delivered my soul from death;
Have you no delivered my feet from stumbling?
That I may walk before God in the light of the living.
(*Psalm 56:12-14*)

Daughter, your faith has made you well. Go in peace, and be healed of your disease. (*Mark 5:34*)

The Lord is my strength and my song
And God has become my salvation. (*Psalm 118:14*)

I shall not die, but live
And declare the works of the Lord. (*Psalm 118:17*)

I love that the Lord should hear
My voice and my supplication.
Because You have inclined Your ear unto me,
Therefore, will I call upon You all my days.
The cords of death compassed me,
And the straits of the nether world got hold of me;
I found trouble and sorrow.
But I called upon the name of the Lord:
"I beseech You, O Lord, deliver my soul."
Gracious is the Lord, and righteous;
Yea our God is compassionate.
The Lord preserves the simple;
I was brought low, and You saved me.
Return, O my soul, unto your rest;
For the Lord has dealt bountifully with you.
For You have delivered my soul from death,
My eyes from tears, and my feet from stumbling.
I shall walk before the Lord in the land of the living.
(*Psalm 116:1-10*)

The cords of Death encompassed me
And the floods of the netherworld assailed me.
The cords of the pit surrounded me.
The snares of death confronted me.
In my distress I called upon the Lord,
And cried out unto my God;
Out of Your temple, You heard my voice.
And my cry came before You into Your ears.
When the earth did shake and quake,
The foundations of the mountains did tremble . . .
You sent from on high, You took me;
You drew me out of the many waters.
You delivered me . . . (*Psalm 18:5-8,17-18*)

They that go down to the sea in ships,
that do business in the great waters-
These saw the works of the Lord,
And God's wonders in the deep.
For God commanded, and raised the stormy wind

Which lifted the waves thereof;
They mounted up to heaven,
And went down to the deeps;
Their souls melted away because of their trouble,
They reeled to and fro
And staggered like a drunken man
And all their wisdom was swallowed up.
They cried out to God in their trouble.
And God brought them out of their distresses.
God made the storm calm,
So that the waves thereof were still.
And God led them to their desired haven.
Let them give thanks unto God for God's mercy. (*Psalm 107:23-31*)

Facing Life-threatening Situations

I am continually with You.
You hold my right hand.
You will guide me with Your counsel, and afterward receive me with glory.
Whom have I in heaven but You?
And besides You I desire none upon earth.
My flesh and my heart fail,
But God is the rock of my heart
And my portion forever. (*Psalm 73:23-29*)

You are my living God who saves
My Rock when grief and sorrow fall,
My banner and my refuge strong
My cup's full portion when I call.
My soul I give into your care,
Asleep, awake, for You are near
And with my soul, my body too,
God is with me, I have no fear.
(Adom Olam-Lord of the Universe-Jewish prayer)

The Lord is my shepherd, I shall not want.
You make me lie down in green pastures.
You lead me beside the still waters.

You restore my soul.
You guide me in the paths of righteousness for Your name's sake.
Yea, though I walk through the valley of the shadow of death,
I will fear no evil; for You are with me;
Your rod and Your staff, they comfort me.
You prepare a table before me in the presence of my enemies;
You have anointed my head with oil. My cup runneth over.
Surely goodness and mercy shall follow me all the days of my life
And I shall dwell in the house of the Lord forever. (*Psalm 23*)

Cast Your burdens upon the Lord and God will sustain you. (*Psalm 55:23*)

God is our refuge and strength, a very present help in trouble.
Therefore, we will not fear. (*Psalm 46:2*)

Save me, O God;
For the waters have come in even unto my soul.
I am sunk deep in mire, where there is no standing.
I am come into deep waters, and the flood overwhelms me.
I am weary with crying; my throat is dried.
My eyes fail while I wait for my God. (*Psalm 69:2-4*)

Deliver me out of the mire,
And let me not sink;
Let me be delivered from them that hate me,
And out of the deep waters.
Let not the flood overwhelm me,
Neither let the deep swallow me up.
And let not the pit shut her mouth upon me.
Answer me, O God, for Your mercy is good. (*Psalm 69:15-17*)

Be faithful unto death, and I will give you the crown of life. (*Revelation 2:10*)

My God, Source of life and death, I turn to You in trust.
Although I pray for life and health, if my life must end soon, let me die, I
pray, in peace. I confess that I have sinned and left much undone, yet I also
know that I have tried to do good. May my acts of goodness redeem my soul,
and may my errors be forgiven. As I ask forgiveness for my sins, I forgive
those who have sinned against me. Protector of the weak and the bereaved,

watch over my loved ones. Into Your hand I commit my spirit; redeem it O God of mercy and compassion.

God reigns; God reigned; God will reign forever and ever.

Our Lord is God.

Hear O Israel the Lord our God the Lord is one.

(adaption of Viddui, the Jewish Final Confession)

After Death of a Loved One

To everything there is a season,
A time to everything under the sun;
A time to be born and a time to die;
A time to laugh and a time to cry
A time to dance and a time to mourn
A time to seek and a time to lose.
This is our time to remember with love
Those whose lives touched ours,
Whose memories will remain with us always.
(adapted from *Ecclesiastes 3*)

So it is with the resurrection of the dead. What is sown is perishable, what is raised is imperishable. It is sown in dishonor, it is raised in glory. It is sown in weakness, it is raised in power. It is sown in a physical body, it is raised a spiritual body. (*I Corinthians 15:42-44*)

Lo! I tell you a mystery. We shall not all sleep, but we shall all be changed, in a moment, in the twinkling of an eye; at the last trumpet. For the trumpet will sound, and the dead will be raised imperishable . . . Then shall come to pass the saying that is written, "Death is swallowed up in victory. O death where is thy victory? O death where is thy sting?" (*I Corinthians 51-52, 54-55*)

When Traveling or Moving

The Lord shall keep you from all evil;
God shall keep your soul.
The Lord shall guard your going out
and your coming in,
from this time forth, and forever. (*Psalm 121:7-8*)

Whither shall I go from Your spirit?
Or whither shall I fell from Your presence?
If I ascend into heaven, You are there;
If I make my bed in the netherworld,
Behold You are there.
If I take the wings of the morning,
And I dwell in the uttermost part of the sea;
Even there You would lead me,
And Your right hand would hold me.
And if I say surely the darkness shall envelop me
And the light about me shall be night;
Even the darkness is not too dark for You
But the night shines as the day;
The darkness is even as the light. (*Psalm 139:7-12*)

When Feeling Guilty or in Need of Forgiveness

Be gracious to me, O God, according to Your mercy;
According to the multitude of Your compassion
Blot out my transgressions.
Wash me thoroughly from my iniquity,
And cleanse me from my sin,
for I know my transgressions,
And my sin is ever before me.
Against You only have I sinned,
And done that which is evil in Your sight. (*Psalm 51:3-6*)

Turn to me and be gracious to me;
For I am solitary and afflicted.
The troubles of my heart are enlarged;
O bring me out of my distresses
See my affliction and my travail;
And forgive all my sins. (*Psalm 25;16-18*)

I acknowledged my sin unto You,
And my iniquity I have not hid;
I said "I will make confession

concerning my transgressions unto the Lord."
And You forgave the iniquity of my sin. (*Psalm 32:5*)

Create me a clean heart, O God;
And renew a steadfast spirit within me.
Cast me not away from Your presence;
And take not Your holy spirit from me.
Restore unto me the joy of Your salvation;
And let a willing spirit uphold me.
Then will I teach transgressors Your ways;
And sinners shall return unto You.
Deliver me from blood-guiltiness, O God,
You God of my salvation.
SO shall my tongue sing aloud of your righteousness.
O Lord open my lips;
And my mouth shall declare Your praise.
For You delight not in sacrifice, else I would give it;
You have no pleasure in burnt offering.
The sacrifices of God are a broken spirit;
A broken and contrite heart, O God, You will not despise. (*Psalm 51:12-19*)

Help us O God to our salvation,
For the sake of the glory of Your name.
And deliver us, and forgive our sins,
For Your name's sake.(*Psalm 79:9*)
Repent for the kingdom of heaven is at hand. (*Matthew 3:17*)

Forgive us our trespasses as we forgive those who trespass against us. And lead us not into temptation but deliver us from evil. For if you forgive men their trespasses, your heavenly Father also will forgive you, but if you do not forgive men their trespasses, neither will your Father forgive your trespasses. (*Matthew 6:12-15*)

Only for God, wait in stillness my soul;
From God comes my salvation.
God only is my rock and my salvation,
My high tower, I shall not be moved.
Upon God rests my salvation and my glory,
The rock of my strength and my refuge is my God.

Trust in God at all times, you people;
Pour out your heart to God;
God is a refuge for us. (*Psalm 62:6-9*)

Thanksgiving

Offer unto God the sacrifice of thanksgiving;
And pay the vows unto The Most High.
And call upon Me in the day of trouble
I will deliver you, and you will honor Me. (*Psalm 50:14-15*)

Whosoever offers the sacrifice of thanksgiving honors Me;
And to him that orders his way aright
Will I show the salvation of God. (*Psalm 50:23*)

O give thanks unto the Lord;
For He is good.
For His mercy endures forever. (*Psalm 106:1*)

Sing unto the Lord with thanksgiving,
Sing praises upon the harp unto our God;
Who covers the heaven with clouds,
Who prepares rain for the earth,
Who makes the mountains to spring with grass. (*Psalm 147:7-8*)

I know that the Lord will
Maintain the cause of the poor,
And the right of the needy.
Surely the righteous shall give
Thanks unto thy name;
The upright shall dwell in Thy presence. (*Psalm 140:13-14*)

O give thanks unto the Lord for He is good,
For His mercy endures forever.
O give thanks unto the Lord of lords
For his mercy endures forever.
To Him alone who does great wonders
For his mercy endures forever.

To Him that by understanding made the heavens
For his mercy is everlasting.
To Him that spread forth the earth above the waters
For his mercy endures forever.
For Him who made great lights;
For his mercy endures forever.
The sun to rule by day
For his mercy endures forever
The moon and the stars to rule by night
For his mercy endures forever. (*Psalm 136: 1-9*)

In Fear

We shall not fear though earth itself should shake,
though the mountains fall into the heart of the sea,
though the waters thunder and rage,
though the winds lift its waves to the very vault of heaven.
We shall not fear, for You are with us;
we shall rejoice in Your deliverance. (adaptation of *Psalm 46*)

The Lord is my light and my salvation,
Who shall I fear?
The Lord is the stronghold of my life;
Of whom shall I be afraid? (*Psalm 27:1*)

I sought the Lord and he answered me,
And delivered me from all my fears." (*Psalm 34:5*)

My heart does writhe within me,
And the terrors of death are fallen upon me.
Fear and trembling come upon me,
And horror has overwhelmed me . . .
But as for me, I will call upon God;
And the Lord will save me. (*Psalm 55:5-6,17*)

Do not fear, only believe. (*Mark 5:36*)

Cast your burden upon the Lord,
And God will sustain you. (*Psalm 55:23*)

Let be and know that I am God. (*Psalm 46:11*)

You shall not be afraid of the terror by night,
Nor of the arrow that flies by day;
Of the pestilence that walks in darkness,
Nor of the destruction that wastes at noonday . . .
You have made the Lord who is my refuge,
Even The Most High, your habitation
There shall no evil befall you
Neither shall any plague come into your tent.
For He will give his angels charge over you
To keep you in all your ways. (*Psalm 91:5-6, 9-11*)

Feeling Lonely, Abandoned, Angry

Why do you stand far off, O Lord?
Why do You hide Yourself in times of trouble. (*Psalm 10:1*)
How long, O Lord, will you forget me forever?
How long will You hide Your face from me?
How long will I take counsel in my soul,
Having sorrow in my heart by day?
Behold, and answer me, O Lord my God;
Lighten my eyes lest I sleep the sleep of death;
Lest my enemies say, "I have prevailed against him;"
Lest my enemies rejoice when I am moved.
But as for me, In Your mercy do I trust.
My heart shall rejoice in Your salvation.
I will sing unto the Lord
because he has dealt bountifully with me. (*Psalm 13*)

My God, my God, why have you forsaken me?
And are far off from my help at the words of my cry.
Oh, my God, I call by day, but You answer not;
And at night, and there is no surcease for me;
Yet You are holy. (*Psalm 22:2-4*)

Alphabet Soup

The staff

PCP Personal Care Physician
NHA Nursing Home administrator
DON Director of Nursing
RHD Registered Dietician
BSW Bachelor's degree in Social Work
MSW Master's degree in Social Work
PT Physical therapy/therapist
OT (also COTA)Occupational therapy/therapist
SPT Speech therapist
ADC-Activity director, certified
CTRS Certified Recreation therapist
RN Registered Nurse
LPN Licensed practical nurse
CNA Certified nurse's aide

The Terms

ABT antibiotic
ABD abdomen
AC before meals
ADL activities of daily living
BID twice daily
BP blood pressure
C/O complains of
DNR do not resuscitate
Dx diagnosis
ECG electrocardiogram
EEG electroencephalogram
ENT Ear, nose, throat
EENT eyes, ear, nose, throat
Fx fracture
H hour
H&P history and physical
HS at bedtime
Hx history (usually medical)

NPO nothing by mouth
NT nasogastric tube
O oxygen
PO by mouth
PER by
PO by mouth
PRN whenever necessary
QD every day
QID four times a day
ROM range of motion
Rx prescription
SOB short of breath
TID three times a day
Tx treatment

The Conditions

AD:	Alzheimer's disease
Agnosis:	inability to correctly identify environmental stimuli
ALS:	Amyotrophic lateral sclerosis (Lou Gehrig's disease)
Aphasia:	partial or complete loss of power to use or understand words
Apraxia:	loss of memory of how to perform complex muscular movement
ASCVD:	arteriosclerotic vascular disease
ASHD:	cardiosclerotic heart disease
Ca:	cancer
CHF:	congestive heart failure
COPD:	chronic obstructive pulmonary disease
CVA:	Cardiovascular accident, stroke
DDD:	degenerative disc disease
Diapheretic:	cold, clammy sweat
DJD:	Degenerative joint disease
Dysphagia:	difficulty with speech and swallowing
HOH:	hard of hear of hearing
IDDM:	insulin dependent diabetes mellitus, type I
MS:	Multiple sclerosis
NIDDM:	noninsulin dependent diabetes mellitus, type II
PAD:	peripheral arterial disease
PD:	Parkinson's disease
PVD:	peripheral vascular disease

SDAT:	Senile dementia, Alzheimer's type
URI:	upper respiratory infection
UTI:	urinary tract infection

Phrases

Activities of Daily Living (ADL): normal everyday actions like dressing, washing, feeding, toileting

Advanced Directives: documents that say who will make medical or legal decisions for you and what treatments you want or don't want if you are incapable of deciding for yourself.

Living Will: a document that says what medical treatments you want or don't want if you can't speak for yourself(e.g. feeding tubes, dialysis, resuscitation, respirator)

Financial Power of Attorney: A document giving someone the right to make financial decisions for you, pay your bills, sign checks if you are mentally or physically incapable of doing so.

Medical Power of Attorney: A document giving someone the right to make medical decisions for you (such as seeing that your Living Will is honored)

DNR: Do not resuscitate. An order that if you stop breathing doctors should not try to shock you back to life. If you do not wish to be resuscitated, a DNR order should be part of your Living Will.

Resident's Rights (These are from Pennsylvania) Contact your local agency on aging to get the ones from your state.

1. The organization addresses ethical issues and respects residents' rights in providing care.
2. The resident is informed of his or her rights before or on admission.
3. Residents are involved in all aspects of their care.
4. Residents are involved in resolving conflicts about care decisions.
5. The resident has a right to a quality of life that supports independent expression, choice, and decision-making, consistent with applicable law and regulation.
6. The resident has a right to considerate care that respects his or her personal values, beliefs, cultural and spiritual preferences, and life-long patterns of living.
7. The resident has a right to personal freedom and dignity.
8. The resident has a right to impartial access to treatment or accommodations.
9. The resident has a right to confidentiality of information.
10. The resident has a right to privacy and security.
11. The resident has a right the exercise citizenship privileges.
12. The resident has a right to unlimited contact with visitors and others.
13. The resident has a right to freedom from chemical or physical restraint.
14. The resident has a right to freedom from mental, physical, sexual or verbal abuse or neglect.
15. The resident has a right to perform or refuse to perform tasks in or for the organization.
16. The resident has a right to participate or refuse to participate in social, spiritual, or community activities and groups.
17. The resident has the right to keep and use personal clothing and possessions.
18. The resident has the right to an environment that ensures dignity and contributes to a positive self-image.
19. The resident has a right to manage or delegate management of personal financial affairs.
20. As appropriate to the care plan, the resident has a right to access transportation services
21. The resident has a right to effective communication.
22. The resident has a right to have complaints heard, reviewed, and, if possible, resolved.
23. The resident has a right to a resident council.

24. The resident has a right to select medical and dental care providers.

25. The resident has a right to purchase medications from a pharmacy of their choice. The pharmacy must enter into a contract ensuring compliance with the facility's policies and procedures regarding pharmacy services. (A copy of policies and procedures will be provided). The facility reserves the right to terminate services of resident-selected pharmacy for non-compliance.

26. The resident has a right to communicate with his medical and dental care providers.

27. The resident has a right to give informed consent.

28. The resident has a right to receive information about advanced directives in order to make informed decisions about providing or withholding heroic measures or resuscitative services and to elect a surrogate if unable to express wishes.

BIBLIOGRAPHY

Albom, Mitch. **Tuesdays with Morrie.** NY: Doubleday, 1997. A Book of wisdom on living from a dying man.

Aranda, Maria et al. **Activity Programming for Persons with Dementia.** Chicago: Alzheimer's Association, 1995, 136 pages. Programming ideas for activities staff dealing with Alzheimer's patients.

Beerman, Susan and Judith Rappaport-Musson. **The Eldercare 911 Question and Answer Book.** Amherst, NY: Prometheus Books, 2005, 304 pages. Questions from caretakers with supportive, informative responses.

Behoref Hayamim, In the Winter of Life: A Values-Based Jewish Guide for Decision Making at the End of Life. Wyncote PA: Reconstructionist Rabbinical College Center for Jewish Ethics, 2002

Beresford, Larry. **The Hospice Handbook**. NY: Little, Brown, 1993
Berman, Claire. **Caring for Yourself While Caring for Your Aging Parents: How to Help, How to Survive**. NY: Henry Holt & Co., 1996

Berrin, Susan, ed. **A Heart of Wisdom: Making the Jewish Journey from Midlife Through the Elder Years.** Woodstock VT. Jewish Lights Publishing, 1997

Bleich, J. David. **Judaism and Healing: Halakhic Perspectives.** KTAV Publishing, 1981

Blidstein, Gerald. **Honor Thy Father and Mother: Filial Responsibility in Jewish Law and Ethics.** NY: KTAV Publishing, 1976

Bowlby, Caroll. **A Comprehensive Text on Alzheimer's and Other Dementias.** Maryland: Aspen Publishing, 1992, 415 pages. Includes programming ideas.

Brener, Anne. **Mourning and Mitzvah: A Guided Journal for Walking the Mourner's Path Through Grief to Healing.** Woodstock VT: Jewish Lights Publishing, 1993

Burger, Sarah Greene. **Nursing Homes: Getting Good Care There.** Atascadero CA: Impact Publishers, 1996

Callanan, Maggie and Patricia Kelley. **Final Gifts: Understanding the Special Awareness, Needs, and Communications of the Dying.** NY: Bantam Books, 1992

Carroll, David. **Living With Dying: A Loving Guide for Family and Close Friends.** St. Paul MN: Paragon House, 1991

Carter, Rosalynn. **Helping Yourself Help Others: A Book for Caregivers.** NY: Random House, 1994.

Cohen Donna and Carl Eisdorfer. **Caring for Your Aging Parents: A Planning and Action Guide.** NY: Tarcher, Putnam, 1995

Collett, Merrill. **Stay Close and Do Nothing: A Spiritual and Practical Guide to Caring for the Dying at Home.** Kansas City MO: Andrews McNeel Publishing, 1997

Davies, Helen and Michael Jensen. **Alzheimer's: The Answers You Need.** Elder Books, 1998

Delehanty, Hugh and Elinor Ginzler. **Caring for Your Parents—A Complete Family Guide: Practical Advice You Can Trust From the Experts at AARP.** AARP, 2008

De Lone, Susan Talia. **Love, Loss & Healing: a Woman's Guide to Transforming Grief.** Portland OR: Sibyl Publications, 1998

Edelman, Hope. **Motherless Daughters: The Legacy of Loss**. NY: Addison-Wesley, 1994.

Ericsson, Stephanie. **Companion Through the Darkness: Inner Dialogues on Grief.** NY: HarperPerennial, 1993

Fein, Leonard. **Against the Dying of the Light: A Father's Journey through Loss.** Woodstock VT: Jewish Lights Publishing, 2001

Freeman, Sally. **Activities and Approaches for Alzheimer's.** 90 pages. Activities staff guide to programming for dementia patients.

Friedman, Rabbi Dayle. **Jewish Pastoral Care: A Practical Handbook from Traditional & Contemporary Sources**. Woodstock VT. Jewish Lights Publishing, 2001. Guide for clergy and staff dealing with Jewish patients.

Frigo, Victoria et al. **You Can Help Someone Who's Grieving: A How-to Healing Handbook.** NY: Penguin Books, 1996

Furman, Joan and David McNabb. **The Dying Time: Practical Wisdom for the Dying & Their Caregivers.** NY: Bell Tower, 1997

Gola, Jitka. Doing Things: **A Guide to Programming for Persons with Alzheimer's Disease and Related Disorders.** Baltimore: Johns Hopkuins Press, 1987, 149 pages. A guide to meaningful programs for dementia patients aimed at activities staff.

Greenberg, Rabbi Sidney. **A Treasury of Comfort**. No. Hollywood CA. Wilshire Book Co., 1954, Readings for comfort and healing.

Gruetzner, Howard. **Alzheimer's: A Caregiver's Guide and Source Book.** NY: Wiley and Son, 2002, 355 pages. Information about caring for Alzheimer's patients and finding helpful resources.

Heath, Angela. **Long Distance Caregiving: A Survival Guide for Far Away Caregivers.** American Source Books, 1991

Hellen, Carly. **Alzheimer's Disease: Activity-focused Care.** Stoneham,MA: Butterworth-Heinemann, 1992, 152 pages. Activities for Alzheimer's patients.

Henry, Stella Mora. **The Eldercare Handbook: Difficult Choices, Compassionate Solutions.** Collins Publishing, 2006, 244 pages.

Hertz, J.H., ed. **The Pentateuch and Haftorahs**, 2nd ed. London: Soncino Press, 1981

Holy Bible. NY: Thomas Nelson Inc., 1972
The Holy Scriptures, Volume II. Philadelphia: The Jewish Publication Society, 1985

Jampolsky, Gerald. **LOVE is Letting Go of Fear.** Berkeley CA: Celestial Arts, 1979

Kasser, Carol. **Cast me Not Off When I am Old.** Lincoln, NE: iUniverse, 2004, 82 pages. The forerunner to this book, with some of the same information.

Kasser, Carol. **Manna for the Soul: Thoughts on Religion and Spirituality.** Lincoln NE: Writers Club Press, 2000

Kasser, Carol. **Reflections: Readings of Spirituality, Gratitude, And Love.** Borders, 2005, 90 pages. Readings of healing and comfort.

Kennedy, Alexandra. **Losing a Parent: Passages to a New Way of Living/ A Guide to Facing Death and Dying.** NY: HarperCollins, 1991

Kenney, Dennis and Elizabeth Oettinger. **The Family Carebook: A Comprehensive Guide for Families of Older Adults.** CAREsource Program Development, 1994

Kolatch, Alfred. **The Jewish Mourner's Book of Why.** NY: Jonathan David Publishers, 1993

Kriseman, Nancy. **The Caring Spirit Approach to Eldercare: A Training Guide for Professionals and Families.** Health Professions Press, 2005, 206 pages.

Kubler-Ross, Elisabeth. **Death: The Final Stage of Growth.** NY: Simon & Schuster, 1975

Kuhn, Daniel. **Alzheimer's Early Stages.** Alameda: Hunter House, 2003, 302 pages.

Kushner, Harold: **When Bad Things Happen to Good People.** NY: Avon, 1981

Lamm, Maurice. **The Jewish Way in Death and Mourning.** NY: Jonathan David Publishers, 1969

Lebow, Grace and Barbara Kane. **Coping With Your Difficult Older Parent: A Guide for Stressed-Out Children.** BarbaraAvon Books, 1999

Lord, Janice Harris. **Beyond Sympathy: What to Say and DO For Someone Suffering an Injury, Illness or Loss.** Ventura CA: Pathfinder Publishing, 1988

Lord, Janice Harris. **No Time for Goodbyes: Coping with Sorrow, Anger and Injustice After a Tragic Death.** Ventura CA: Pathfinder Publishing, 1987

Lotvig, Jytte and John Becker. **Alzheimer's A to Z.** Oakland: New Harbinger Publishing, 1999, 25 pages. A comprehensive guide to dealing with Alzheimer's patients.

Loverde, Joy. **The Complete Eldercare Planner: Where to Start, Questions to Ask and How to Find Help.** Hyperion, 1997

A Loving Voice: A Caregiver's Book of Read-aloud Stories for the Elderly. Philadelphia: Charles Press, 1992, 293 pages. Wonderful stories to tap into childhood memories of elders.

Lustbader, Wendy and Nancy Hooyman. **Taking Care of Aging Family Members: A Practical Guide**. NY: Simon & Schuster, 1994

Mace, Nancy and Peter Robins. **The 36-Hour Day: A Family Guide to Caring for Persons with Alzheimer's Disease, Related Dementia, Illness and Memory Loss at Later Life.** Johns Hopkins University Press, 1991, 586 pages.

Marcell, Jacqueline. **Elder Rage or Take My Father . . . Please: How to Survive Caring for Aging Parents**. Irvine CA: Impressive Press, 2000. Dealing with anger in aging parents.

Matthews, Joseph. **Beat the Nursing Home Trap: A Consumer's Guide to Choosing & Financing Long-Term Care.** Nolo Self-Help Law, 1993

McEldowney, James. **God's Presence Among the Aging: 55 Meditations for Seniors.** Bradenton FL: The Southmark Foundation of Gerontology, 1988.

McGowin Diana Friel. **Living in the Labyrinth: A Personal Journey through the maze of Alzheimer's**. NY: Delacorte Press, 1993

McLeod, Beth Witrogen. **Caregiving: The Spiritual Journey of Love, Loss and Renewal.** John Wiley & Sons, 1999

The Merck Manual of Health and Aging. NY: Ballantine Books, 2004, 951 pages.

Metrick, Sydney Barbara. **Crossing the Bridge: Creating Ceremonies for Grieving and Healing From Life's Losses**. Berkley CA: Celestial Arts, 1994

Meyer, Maria and Paul Derr. **The Comfort of Home: An Illustrated Step-by-Step Guide for Caregivers.** CareTrust Publications, 1998

Morris, Virginia. **How to Care for Aging Parents. NY:** Workman Publishing, 2004, 685 pages.

Myerhoff, Barbara. **Number Our Days.** NY: Simon & Schuster, 1978. Lovingly-told stories about members of a California senior center.

Olitzky, Rabbi Kerry. **Jewish Paths toward Healing and Wholeness.** Woodstock VT: Jewish Lights Publishing, 2000

Orenstein, Rabbi Deborah, ed. **Lifecycles: Jewish Women on Life Passages and Personal Milestones,** Volume 1. Woodstock, VT: Jewish Lights Publishing, 1994

Pipher, Mary. **Another Country: Navigating the Emotional Terrain of Our Elders.** NY: Riverhead Books, 2004, 208 pages.

Polish, Daniel. **Bringing the Psalms to Life**. Woodstock VT: Jewish Lights Publishing, 2000

Radin, Lisa and Gary, eds. **What if it's Not Alzheimer's?** NY: Prometheus, 2005, 328 pages. Defines the differences between various dementias, offers advice for caregivers, and suggests some programming ideas.

Raphael, Simcha Paul. **Jewish View of the Afterlife.** Northvale NJ: Jason Aronson, Inc., 1996

Riemer, Jack and Nathaniel Stampfer, eds. **Ethical Wills: A Modern Jewish Treasury.** NY: Schocken Books, 1983

Rinpoche, Sogyal. **The Tibetan Book of Living and Dying**. NY: HarperCollins, 1992

Sankar, Andrea. **Dying at Home: A Family Guide to Caregiving.** Johns Hopkins University press, 1991

Sarna, Nahum. **On the Book of Psalms: Exploring the Prayers of Ancient Israel.** NY: Schocken Books, 1993

Schacter-Shalomi, Zalman and Ronald Miller. **From Age-ing to Sage-ing: A profound New Vision of Growing Older.** NY: Warner Books, 1995

Siegel, Bernie, M.D. **Love, Medicine & Miracles: Lessons Learned About Self-Healing from a Surgeon's Experience With Exceptional Patients**. NY: Harper& Row, 1986

Silverman, William and Kenneth Cinnamon. **When Mourning Comes: A Book of Comfort for the Grieving.** Northvale NJ: Jason Aronson, 1990

Sonsino, Rifat and Daniel Syme. **What Happens After I Die?: Jewish Views of Life After Death.** NY: UAHC Press, 1990

Straus, Livia Selmanowitz. **A Flickering Candle: Death and End of Life Issues**. United Synagogue of Conservative Judaism, 1994.

Strauss, Claudia. **Talking to Alzheimer's**. Oakland: New Harbinger Publishing, 161 pages.

Susik, D. Helen. **Hiring Home Caregivers: The Family Guide to In-Home Eldercare.** Atascadero CA: Impact Publishers/American Source Books

Taylor, Dan. **The Parent Care Conversation**. NY: Penguin Group, 2006, 262 pages. Useful guide for helping families help their parents make preparations for their elder years.

Taylor, Kylea. **The Ethics of Caring: Honoring the Web of Life in Our Professional Healing Relationships**. Santa Cruz CA: Hanford Mead Publishers, 1995

Visiting Nurses Association of America. **Caregiver's Handbook: A Complete Guide to Home Health Care.** DK Publishing, 1998

Wall, Kathleen and Gary Ferguson. **Rites of Passage: Celebrating Life's Changes.** Hillsboro OR: Beyond Words Publishing, 1998

Warner, Mark. **The Complete Guide to Alzheimer's-Proofing Your Home.** Purdue University Press, 1998

Weintraub, Rabbi Simkha. **Healing of Soul, Healing of Body: Spiritual Leaders Unfold the Strength and Solace in Psalms.** Woodstock VT: Jewish Lights Publishing, 1994

Westberg, Granger. **Good Grief.** Philadelphia: Fortress Press, 1962

Whitfield, Barbara Harris. Final **Passage: Sharing the Journey as This Life Ends.** Deerfield Beach FL: Health Communications Inc., 1998

Williams, Gene and Kay Patie. **The Caregiver's Manual: A Guide to Helping the Elderly and Infirm.** Citadel Press, 1995

Zukerman, Rachelle. **Elder Care for Dummies.** NY: Wiley Publishing, 2003, 354 pages. A fact-filled but impersonal presentation of information on caring for elders.

ON-LINE RESOURCES

www.aahsa.org The American Association of Homes and Services for the Aging provides information about alternate housing communities for seniors.

www.AARP.org Information on health, leisure, insurance issues for people 55 and older

www.AgingUSA.com Helpful information and resources for age-related issues.

www.ahaf.com The American Health Assistance Foundation provides information on Alzheimer's and Macular Degeneration.

www.alz.org The Alzheimer's Association website provides information about all aspects of Alzheimer's issues.

www.alzheimers.org The website of the Alzheimer's Disease Education and Referral Center provides information and referral options for Alzheimer's patients and caregivers.

www.ama-assn.org has a physician locator service. Use the *Doctor Finder* prompt and the specialty *geriatrics* to find doctors specializing in care for seniors

www.aoa.gov The Administration on Aging, part of the Department of Health and Human Services, provides services and resources for the elderly and family caregivers.

www.apdaparkinson.org Information about Parkinson's disease.

www.aplaceformom.com A free referral service for families looking for senior care option.

www.arthritis.org Information in Spanish and English on arthritis-related issues.

www.asaging.org. The American Society on Aging provides information, education, and resources to all professionals dealing with the physical, emotional, spiritual, social, and economic aspects of aging.

www.bartonmedical.com Barton Medical equipment provides pictures and specific product details of equipment that allows one person to secure and safely transfer patients.

www.benefitscheckup.org Finds programs for people 55 and older that help with expenses for prescriptions, healthcare, utilities, and other essentials. It can help elders identify benefits they did not know they were entitled to.

www.booksaloud.org Provides free audio book services.

www.cahcinc.org The Center to Advance Hospice Care promotes hospice awareness, gives free educational programs, and helps find hospice programs in the greater Philadelphia area and surrounding suburbs.

www.cancer.org The American Cancer Society website provides information on research and treatment for cancer.

www.cancercare.org Information on cancer treatments and research.

www.caps4caregivers.org Networking and information for children of aging parents.

www.caregiver.org provides information, services, research and advocacy for family caregivers.

www.caregivermall.com. Has free information on eldercare and age-related illnesses.

www.caregiverpartnership.com sells products for incontinence, nutritional, diabetic, wound care, daily living, personal care and arthritis needs.

www.caremanager.org The National Association of Professional Geriatric Care Managers provides addresses for geriatric care managers throughout the United States who can help elder clients and their families with counseling, treatment, and services.

www.carepathways.com is a site run by RNs to provide care information to seniors and their families.

www.carf.org/aging Information about accreditation standings of Continuing Care facilities

www.caring.com provides Boomers caring for elderly parents with medical, legal, financial and nutritional information

www.caringtoday.com Practical advice for family caregivers

www.cms.gov A government website for Medicare and Medicaid Services provides consumers and professionals with current information on Medicare, Medicaid and related programs.

www.crossroadshospice.com Supports patients, families, and healthcare professionals dealing with end-of-life issues.

www.eldercare.gov The Eldercare Locator provides information for older adults and caregivers including an extensive glossary, caregiver resources, and referrals to local services.

www.elderweb.com This site provides links to eldercare services in different states and countries.

www.healthfinder.gov The federal healthfinder website including a health library and provides information for caregivers and healthcare professionals on long-term care and insurance issues.

www.healthinaging.org This the website of the American geriatrics Society.

www.helpingpatients.org Website of Pharmaceutical Research and Manufacturers of America assists patients in finding programs to help them get their medications.

www.homecareofpa.com Information of home health care in Philadelphia.

www.hospice-america.org Contains information and links to sources related to various aspects of hospice care.

www.infoaging.org. Information on the biology of aging and common age-related ailments.

www.link-to-life.com Link To Life provides personal emergency response services to the sick and elderly nationwide.

www.mayohealth.org The Mayo Clinic's website includes a Healthy Aging Center that provides information on medical conditions, diet, exercise, stress reduction, risk avoidance, physical, mental, and emotional health.

www.medicare.gov Provides information about Medicare and Medicaid nursing homes in the United States.

www.medicareadvocacy.org Center for Medicare Advocacy has information on Medicare coverage and health care for elders and people with disabilities.

www.naccm.net. The National Academy of Certified Care Managers requires its members to pass a standardized examination to assure the professional skills of care managers.

www.naela.com The National Academy of Elder Law Attorneys provides addresses of lawyers throughout the United States who work with seniors regarding benefits, probate, estate planning and guardianship, healthcare, advance directives, and long-term planning.

www.ncoa.org The National Council on the Aging provides resources, information and advocacy on issues of health, safety, relationships as well as help with utility, medical and prescription costs.

www.n4a.org The National Association of Area Agencies on Aging provides information on services and advocacy for the elderly.

www.parkinson.org The National Parkinson's Foundation provides information and medical support related to Parkinson's disease.

www.society-csa.com The CSA educates insurance, accounting, law, clergy, health, real estate, and other professionals to understand needs of seniors in areas of housing, health, and estate planning.

www.ssa.gov The Social Security Administration's website answers questions and provides information on Social Security benefits including applications for retirement, disability, and survivor benefits.

www.stroke.org The National Stroke Association provides information and referrals related to strokes.

www.strokeassociation.org Information for stroke victims and their caregivers.

www.thefamilycaregiver.org The National Family Caregivers Association provides news, information and advocacy for family caregivers.

www.thirdage.com Issues of health and relationships for people in midlife

www.va.gov The Department of Veteran Affairs provides information on benefits, and services including healthcare, pension, and burial for qualified veterans.

www.whenourparents.com/forum Networking site for caregivers